GW00372804

HEART HEALTH

A SELF-HELP GUIDE

COMBINING ORTHODOX AND COMPLEMENTARY APPROACHES TO HEALTH

HEADWAY HEALTHWISE

HEART HEALTH

A SELF-HELP GUIDE
COMBINING ORTHODOX AND COMPLEMENTARY APPROACHES TO HEALTH

HASNAIN WALJI & DR ANDREA KINGSTON

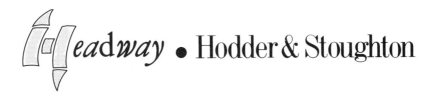

Headway • Hodder & Stoughton

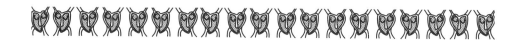

Cataloguing in Publication Data is available from the British Library

ISBN 0 340 60562 6

First published 1994
Impression number 10 9 8 7 6 5 4 3 2 1
Year   1998 1997 1996 1995 1994

Copyright © 1994 Hasnain Walji

All rights reserved. No part of this publication may be reproduced in any form or by any means, electronic or mechanical, including photocopy, recording, or any information storage and retrieval system, without permission in writing from the publisher or under licence from the Copyright Licensing Agency Limited. Further details of such licences (for reprographic reproduction) may be obtained from the Copyright Licensing Agency Limited, of 90 Tottenham Court Road, London W1P 9HE.

Printed in Great Britain for Hodder & Stoughton Educational, a division of Hodder Headline Plc, 338 Euston Road, London NW1 3BH by Page Bros (Norwich) Ltd.

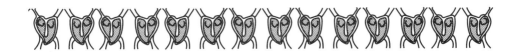

CONTENTS

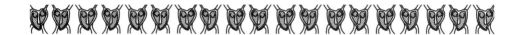

*This book is dedicated to the seekers of health
and to those who help them find it.*

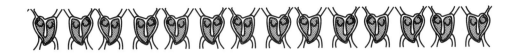

ACKNOWLEDGEMENTS

I should like to express my gratitude to Dr Andrea Kingston for her valuable input and the enlightened way she dealt with a number of apparent contradictions between orthodox medicine and complementary therapies; to nutritionist Angela Dowden for offering many pertinent suggestions; to Sato Liu of the Natural Medicines Society for her assistance in providing contacts and arranging interviews with practitioners; and to my agent Susan Mears for her encouragement and practical help.

This book could not possibly have been written without the co-operation of the following practitioners who have so willingly endured my interruptions: aromatherapy – Christine Wildwood; naturopathy – Jan De Vries; homoeopathy – Michael Thompson and Beth MacEoin; reflexology – Pauline Wills; and anthroposophical medicine – Dr Maurice Orange.

I must thank my daughter Sukaina for giving her time during vacation from university for wading through research papers and books and extracting relevant information. Last but not least, I wish to thank my wife Latifa whose gentle care and concern, not to mention long hours typing the manuscript, enabled me to complete this book.

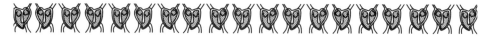

Foreword To The Series
from the Natural Medicines Society

When we visit our doctor's surgery and are given a diagnosis, we often receive a prescription at the same time. More people than ever are now aware that there may be complementary treatments available and would like to explore the possibilities, but do not know which kind of treatment would be most useful for their problem.

There are books on just about every treatment available, but few which start from this standpoint: the patient interested in knowing the options for treating their particular condition – which treatment is available or useful, what the treatment involves, or what to expect when consulting the practitioner.

The Headway Healthwise series will provide the answers for those wishing to consider what treatment is available, once the doctor has diagnosed their condition. Each book will cover both the orthodox and complementary approaches. Although patients are naturally most interested in relieving their immediate symptoms, the books show how complementary treatment goes much deeper; underlying causes are explored and the patient is treated as a whole.

It is important to stress that it is not the intention of this series to replace the expertise of the doctors and practitioners, nor to encourage self-treatment, but to show the options available to the patient.

As the consumer charity working for freedom of choice in medicine, the Natural Medicines Society welcomes the Headway Healthwise series. Although the Natural Medicines Society does not recommend people who are taking prescribed orthodox medicines to stop doing so, our aim is to introduce them to complementary forms of treatment. We believe the orthodox system of medicine is often best used as a last, not first, resort when other, gentler, methods fail or are inappropriate.

Giving patients the information to make their choice is the purpose of this series. With the increasing use of complementary medicine within the NHS, knowing the complementary options is vital both to the patients and to their doctors in the search for better health care.

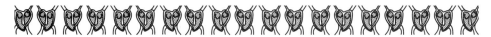

Foreword To The Book

Great Britain is the second worst country in the developed world after Finland for the high number of heart attacks resulting in premature death.

I gave up smoking when I was 10 years old because, as my palate developed, I found that things simply tasted wrong for the 24 hours after even a few puffs. But for those who do smoke, giving up is the single most important intervention they can make to help preserve a long life and a healthy heart.

The money saved can be best spent on increasing the number of portions of fresh fruit and vegetables in the diet to at least five a day, cutting down on red meat and saturated fats, cutting out trans- or hydrogenated fats such as those found in most margarines, eating fatty fish, using garlic and enjoying good bread, olive oil and a few glasses of, preferably red, wine.

But what to do when things go wrong? *Heart Health* provides a lot of the answers in an all-embracing approach that is most refreshing. Earlier this year (1994) I gave a talk to the All Parties Parliamentary Forum on Complementary Medicine in the House of Lords and was able to say that there was a great coming together between experienced practitioners, both orthodox and complementary. An understanding is being reached that there is only one sort of medicine that the patient deserves and that is good medicine. Neither side has a monopoly and each can contribute much to the other. A surgeon once told me that he often used the services of the alternative practitioners in the town where his hospital was situated. When asked how did he know which ones to choose, he replied that that was easy, he chose the ones which came to him when they had problems!

Heart Health epitomises this approach, giving the enquiring reader a glimpse into many different methods of helping the heart and giving good advice as to where reliable practitioners of the various healing arts can be located.

I commend this approach to a wide audience who I hope will gain health, happiness and years by putting into practice some of the ideas so effectively described in the pages that follow.

Maurice Hanssen
Author of *E for Additives*
Ex Chairman and now Patron of the Natural Medicines Society
July 1994

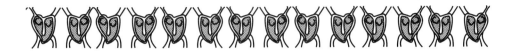

PREFACE

Headway Healthwise is a concise new series which takes the original approach of looking at common ailments and describing how they may be treated using complementary therapies. The aim of the series is not to replace the orthodox medical approach but to give readers an overview of how they may be helped by consulting complementary practitioners.

Once a condition has been diagonised by a GP, those wishing to avail themselves of other forms of treatment will find this book particularly useful. The intention of this series is not to recommend people taking prescribed orthodox medicines to stop taking these. It is to introduce them to alternative and complementary forms of treatment which may enable them reduce the amount of orthodox prescriptions, at the very least, and, in many cases, do away with their need altogether.

We have attempted to present the information in a style that is clear and easy to read. The central approach is to look at addiction from different perspectives by providing you with descriptions of several complementary therapies. While cautioning against self-medication, the book has been written to encourage you to take charge of your own health by making an informed choice of therapy. It shows how and why orthodox medicine – a life-saving and useful system of medicine – should be used as a last resort when other more natural methods fail, rather than the first recourse.

An overview of heart health in the opening chapter is followed by a chapter on the kind of treatment to expect from your GP. The second chapter deals with such factors as lifestyle, diet and nutrition in the management of the disorder. Later chapters look at complementary approaches to the subject.

The one common factor that underpins all the alternative or complementary therapeutic techniques described in this book is the belief in the healing power of the body. Practitioners recognise that the body possesses an inherent ability to cure itself. This gives a clear message to the patient of his/her role in the healing process – that of the mind willing the body to heal itself.

At first sight this may appear to challenge the approach of orthodox medicine, in which the therapeutic objective is to cure the diseased part of the body. The patient has no role to play except dutifully to take the medicine. The concept of a white-coated god who possesses the magic pill to cure is the result of fear combined with a lack of understanding of the nature of disease and, more so, that of health.

This book is an attempt to dispel myths and to bring about a greater understanding of the issues relating to health and healing, which go beyond the realms of simple anatomy and biology. The recognition that orthodox medicine and complementary therapies need not be mutually exclusive, as both have a role to play, can go a long way towards promoting the integrated medicine of the twenty-first century.

Hasnain Walji
Milton Keynes
March, 1994

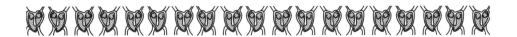

Note: Information given in this book is not intended to be taken as a replacement for medical advice. Any person worried about their health should consult a medical professional. Heart disease can be extremely serious and anyone worried about their heart should consult their GP.

OVERVIEW: YOUR HEART IN YOUR HANDS

If you work too hard, have little time for relaxation or exercise, eat a diet mainly of refined foods, consume large amounts of fats, and are constantly under stress, you are a prime candidate for heart disease. If it is any consolation, you are not alone. This description fits a large majority of our population. Small wonder, then, that the UK is top of the league of nations in the Western world plagued by this disease of modern civilisation. In the UK over 3,000 people die prematurely of heart disease every week. In addition to the immeasurable amount of human misery and suffering, 35 million working days are lost every year, and it costs the NHS £500 million each year in hospital beds (5,000 beds at any one time) and expensive by-pass and heart transplant operations.

The good news is that this killer disease can be avoided. Unlike smallpox, polio or cholera, medical science does not have to discover a *vaccine* (a substance used for inoculation against disease) or an *antibiotic* (a substance used against infections) or a wonder cure to save us from it. It can largely be prevented, and in some cases even reversed, by changes in our lifestyle, diet and stress control.

The health professionals, orthodox and complementary, exhort us in unison to give up smoking, avoid alcohol, eat nutrient-rich foods which are low in refined sugars, fats and salt, exercise regularly and learn to control stress. All these are deciding factors in maintaining heart health and to continue to ignore this advice is to court heart disease.

In 1989 the Government published *The Health of the Nation*, which sets out the targets and objectives for the nation's health to be reached by the year 2000. It covers many aspects of health from food safety to breast-feeding and mental health. *The Health of the Nation* lists coronary heart disease as one of the major causes of death in this country: in 1989, 26 per cent of all deaths were from heart-related diseases. This is an unacceptably and needlessly high level, since most heart disease is preventable. This book is about how you can look after your heart so that you can avoid heart diseases.

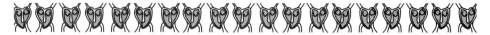

For Heart, Read Arteries

Strictly speaking, the term 'heart disease' is a misnomer. It is not the heart that needs looking after as much as the arteries. We must recognise that our arteries are more than just pipes which carry blood through the body. To maintain good heart health our arteries must be kept in a state where there is no blockage, or hindrance, for blood flow. If our arteries narrow because of unwanted deposits (*atherosclerosis*), the heart has to pump harder to move the blood around the body. If the arteries feeding a part of the heart are blocked because of a blood clot, blood is prevented from reaching the heart and a heart attack then occurs. In the same way, if the arteries feeding the brain are blocked, a stroke occurs. To keep the blood circulation at its optimum it is important that all the factors which cause the arteries to narrow or clots to form are addressed.

Before discussing the factors which improve our heart health and those which undermine it, it is worth taking a little time to look at the heart to understand how it functions.

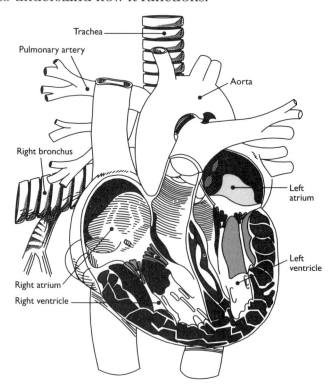

Structure of the heart

How Your Heart Works

The heart is a muscled organ which pumps blood around the body. Over the course of an average lifetime the heart pumps (contracts) 2,500 million times. The frequency and force of each contraction are naturally evolved to produce a healthy circulation depending on the individual and the individual's activity at any given time: athletics, for example, place a much greater demand on the heart than sitting in a chair reading a book. When we talk of 'bad circulation' we mean that the heart is not pumping the blood as efficiently as it could: the result is a feeling of numbed limbs and cold feet.

The heart is made of a special sort of muscle: it is called the *myocardium muscle*. Blood which does not have any oxygen comes into the heart from the top right-hand side, passes down through to the bottom of the heart and is pumped up the heart to exit via the top left-hand side of the heart. From there it flows into the lungs where carbon dioxide passes out of the blood and oxygen enters. The re-oxygenated blood then passes back into the heart. Hence the description *circulatory system*. The heart has valves to ensure that blood circulates in only one direction.

How the heart works

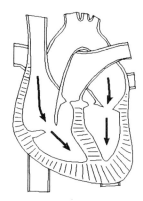

Phase 1: Diastole – resting

Heart fills with blood. Deoxygenated blood flows into the right side of the heart while oxygenated blood flows into the left side.

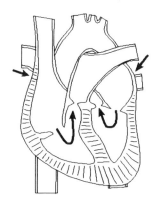

Phase 2: Atrial systole – contraction

The upper chambers (the atria) contract simultaneously, squeezing more blood into the lower chambers (the ventricles), which become full.

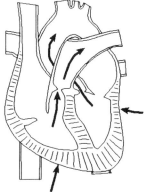

Phase 3: Ventricular systole – contraction

The lower chambers contract to pump deoxygenated blood into the aorta. As soon as the heart is empty, the first phase (diastole) begins again.

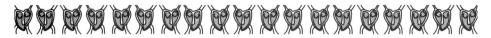

To accommodate the blood flow, the heart has four chambers, an upper and a lower on both the left and right sides. The upper chamber is called the *atrium* and the lower is called the *ventricle*. The heart responds to physical activity in two ways. Firstly, during exercise, such as running, the heart muscle reacts automatically to the demands of the body's muscles for more oxygen by increasing its output, thus stepping up its contraction rate. Secondly, the *autonomic nervous system* plays its part. This controls automatic body responses, for example, the action of the eyes' pupils which widen or contract according to the sensory stimulation they receive. The autonomic nervous system has two effects: increasing activity (described as the *sympathetic nervous system*) and slowing down activity (described as the *parasympathetic nervous system*). The autonomic nervous system can therefore increase the heart rate or decrease it.

When the heart is resting, the average heart rate is between 60 and 100 heartbeats per minute. Very fit people, such as athletes, will have a lower resting rate: this is because the heart works so efficiently it does not need as many contractions to pump the blood around the body. The maximum acceptable heart rate is about 200 beats per minute.

Although the heart continually pumps blood, it does not take its own oxygen requirements from the blood which it is circulating. Instead, two *coronary arteries* supply the heart with its oxygen and nutrient requirements. Each of the main coronary arteries has a network of *arterioles*, small blood vessels, and *capillaries*, even smaller blood vessels, branching off the arterioles.

Factors Which Maintain Cardiovascular Function

The blood supplied to the heart via the coronary arteries must contain sufficient oxygen and nutrients for the heart to function properly. In addition, to carry out its job, the heart needs a sufficient supply of blood through its chambers. For this to be in order, the blood must be able to pass through the body's arteries.

Exercise is paramount to good cardiovascular health – without it, a sluggish circulation, high resting pulse and weakened muscles will result. An avoidance of damaging substances, such as nicotine, hard drugs and cholesterol-rich foods, will avoid the clogging up of the arteries and raised blood pressure.

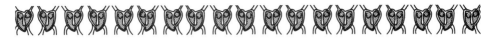

Factors Which Impair Cardiovascular Health

Furring-up The Arteries

In the same way as furred-up plumbing carries less water, unwanted deposits on the artery walls narrow the arteries and hence impair the flow of blood. This is called *atherosclerosis* and is one of the most common causes of coronary heart disease. The word 'atherosclerosis' comes from the Greek word *athera* meaning 'gruel', an apt description of these deposits.

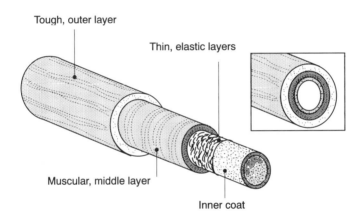

Structure of a healthy artery

Arteries are strong and flexible to carry the pressure of blood flow. They consist of a tough outer lining, a muscular middle layer which allows for minute contraction when blood flow increases and an inner coat – the 'wall' of the artery.

The deposits which can build-up on the inner wall are mainly fats, but also cells from the artery wall itself, tissue and clumps of blood platelets. Unless action is taken, the build-up of deposits will eventually impede blood flow and lead to atherosclerosis, eventually leading to a heart attack.

What Causes Atherosclerosis?

There is a great deal of controversy regarding this and the subject is more complex than appears on the surface. Experts believe that first

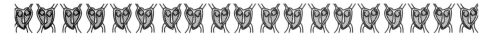

our artery walls are damaged by oxidation then, in an attempt to repair that damage, there is a proliferation of cells in the artery wall which in turn attract *cholesterol* – the *saturated fat* found in animal fats, eggs and dairy products – and other fats, as well as calcium. The excess of any of these exacerbates the furring.

Although cholesterol is required by the body for some of its functions, our Western diets overload us with an excess to such an extent that the body cannot eliminate it; it stays in the body and its stickiness means it attaches firmly to artery walls. But food choices can actually dissolve cholesterol and we shall look at these in Chapter 3.

Sometimes, though, it is through no fault of our diet that disease is present; an inherited ailment such as *diabetes*, which is a disease of the metabolic system, will also aggravate the likelihood of atherosclerosis. Again, attention to diet and lifestyle will reduce the risk of atherosclerosis or a heart attack.

If you think you may have a high cholesterol level, due to your food choices or a metabolic disease, your cholesterol level can be easily measured from a blood sample. Your doctor or health clinic will do this for you.

Smoking

According to *The Health of the Nation*, smoking causes 20 per cent of all coronary heart disease deaths in this country. Any good health-care plan, not just for cardiovascular health, must therefore include stopping, or not starting, smoking.

Nicotine is both a relaxant and a stimulant. As a stimulant it increases the production of the hormone adrenaline which passes into the blood, increasing the heart rate. Tobacco tar releases the gas carbon monoxide, which is poisonous to our bodies. The carbon monoxide released from smoking combines with *haemoglobin* (the molecule which carries oxygen in the blood cells) and interferes with the natural oxygenation in the body. Long-term exposure to carbon monoxide hardens the arteries – again with the effect of reducing the blood flow to the heart. Nicotine also increases the *metabolic rate* (the chemical and physical changes that take place in the body): this means that food is absorbed more quickly and its energy value extracted. This in turn forces the rest of the body to speed up its processes and with it the circulatory system must pump blood around the body faster to keep up.

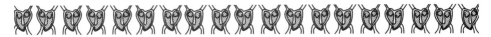

Blood Pressure

The pressure exerted by blood flow through the arteries rises and falls as the heart responds to different activities, such as exercise or stress. Abnormally high pressure is known as *hypertension* and low pressure as *hypotension*.

Low Blood Pressure

Hypotension, the medical term for low blood pressure, can cause cardiovascular problems because the blood pressure is too low for the body's optimum functioning. This is why sufferers of hypotension experience dizziness and fainting, particularly when there is sudden movement.

High Blood Pressure

Hypertension, or high blood pressure, is a high-risk factor in cardiovascular ailments. The blood pressure is too high and strains the heart as it attempts to deal with the rapid flow of blood. Over a long period of time, the heart increases its mass in an attempt to deal with the overload: this raises the heart's requirement for its own blood supply, and as yet autopsies on heart-attack victims do not show correspondingly increased cardiovascular arteries.

Fortunately, hypertension can often be eased through careful attention to its causative factors, such as:

- stress and behaviour patterns;
- lifestyle;
- weight;
- smoking;
- alcohol and salt consumption.

Some people, however, may be following perfectly healthy lifestyles but will have inherited hypertension.

Stress And Behaviour Patterns

We experience stress every day. Its onset can be due to a variety of factors in the home or at work; other people can put us under stress, or we can put ourselves under stress. The effect of stress is to increase our heartbeat, releasing adrenaline, to prepare us for a 'fight or flight' response, all of which places a strain on the heart.

It is not stress itself which is a problem, but how we cope with it. Some people seem to crumple at the slightest difficulty, whilst others can cope with seemingly inordinate amounts of stress. To improve your cardiovascular health, effective stress relief is paramount.

There are also definite types of behaviour which predispose us to stress. Scientists have labelled these as 'Type A' and 'Type B' behaviour. Type A behaviour is associated with people who are always pushing themselves to the limit, always in a rush even when they do not need to be, constantly busy, never sitting still or allowing themselves to relax. Indeed, they regard relaxation as a waste of time. Type A people expect those around them to behave in the same way as themselves. These people are often very ambitious, and unfortunately their constant drive is setting them up for coronary disorders. It is believed that, of men under 60 years of age suffering a heart attack, 90 per cent are Type A personalities.

In contrast, Type B personalities are easy going, calm and find it easy to relax. They are considerate of other people and enjoy life. They are not likely to be fiercely ambitious. Research has found that, even though Type B personalities may smoke and not exercise, they are far less likely to suffer a heart attack.

Weight/Obesity

Obesity increases blood pressure and cholesterol levels and thus the chances of a stroke. Weight loss is of paramount importance to lessen the strain on the heart. If a person is obese through overeating, it is likely that the foods consumed are high in fat and sugar (cakes, biscuits, chocolate, fizzy drinks and so on) but low in nutrients (vitamins and minerals). Combined with exercise, a change of diet to one that does not leave a person feeling hungry but provides the body with the goodness it needs will improve health as well as causing the pounds to fall off. However, thin people suffer from coronary heart disease too.

Chapter 3 will highlight dietary considerations for a healthy heart. It is important to note that even after a heart attack lifestyle and nutritional measures can go a long way to minimise the impact of the attack.

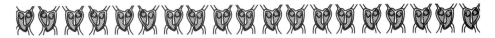

Heart Disorders

Angina Pectoris

Angina is a pain felt in the chest. It can recur frequently without leading to a heart attack. It is a warning symptom that the cardiovascular system is under stress and needs immediate attention.

Angina occurs because insufficient oxygen is reaching the heart. This may be due to stress, atherosclerosis, lack of exercise, smoking or, in rare cases, severe *anaemia*, when there are insufficient red blood cells in the body to carry oxygen.

The chest pain can occur after a meal, during hot temperatures or during stressful periods – in other words, whenever stress is placed on the heart. A medical examination will look to discover the underlying cause of angina and suitable treatment will be accordingly prescribed.

Nutritional Disorders

A lack of nutrients (vitamins and minerals) and protein will damage the heart's health. Instead of being a healthy organ which is effective and strong enough to pump the blood, it will become flabby and weak. Attention to nutrition is of paramount importance.

Arrhythmia

Arrhythmia is an oddity in the heartbeat. It may mean a regular, but slower than safe or faster than safe heartbeat, or an irregular heartbeat. In the case of the latter, a *pacemaker* can be fitted to regulate the heartbeat. Arrhythmia is a symptom of cardiovascular problems, although it is more common after a heart attack – although most people have experienced palpitations. If arrhythmia is suspected, a doctor would measure the heart beat using an ECG (*electrocardiogram*) which measures the electrical impulses of the heart and give treatment accordingly. Attention to diet, blood pressure and stress relief will undoubtedly feature in treatment, and drugs may be required to settle the heartbeat as an immediate action.

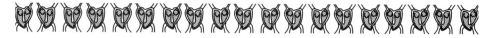

Ischaemic Heart Disease

Ischaemia is the condition when insufficient blood is reaching an organ. In the case of cardiovascular health, this is likely to be due to the narrowing of the coronary arteries.

Myocardial Infarction

Myocardial infarction is the medical term for a heart attack. A sudden pain is felt as the heart seizes up and fails. The pain may be in the chest, down the left arm or, more rarely, in the abdomen. Up to 50 per cent of heart attack sufferers do not survive 20 days after the attack. A mild heart attack can be survived, although damage to the heart may be sustained.

Myocarditis

A viral infection can inflame the heart muscle: this is myocarditis. It usually accompanies an infection of the lungs or *rheumatic fever* (a disease which is characterised by inflammation and pain in the joints).

Heart Defects

These are defects in the heart which occur at birth. They affect the heart chambers, valves or main blood vessels and usually the cure is surgery.

Heart Block

This is a disorder of the electrical impulses which govern the heartbeat. The heartbeat is consequently very slow (40–50 beats per minute); fainting attacks are likely to provide the first indication that all is not well. Diagnosis using an ECG will lead to the fitting of a pacemaker.

Tumours

Heart tumours are rare, but can occur within the heart's chambers. If the tumour is large, it will interfere with the heart's electrical impulses with the result that *arrhythmia*, the irregularity

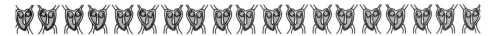

of the heart beat, or *palpitations*, the awareness of a fast heartbeat, will occur. Treatment may be required in the form of surgery to remove the tumour, or drugs to kill it.

Heart Failure

This is not the same as a heart attack, nor as life-threatening. It is usually a case of left-sided or right-sided heart failure, and literally means that that part of the heart has difficulty in functioning. Heart failure is easily treated and patients survive for many years, given correct attention to diet and lifestyle.

Exercise And Heart Health

One way of reducing the risk of heart disease is to lead a more active life. This does not mean becoming a fitness freak. Exercising just a few times a week for 15–20 minutes will ensure a healthier heart.

The heart is a muscle and like the other muscles in in your body it can become weak if it is not sufficiently exercised. Physical fitness enables your heart to deliver enough oxygen through the blood stream to your muscles. Your muscles use this oxygen to provide enough energy to sustain daily activity. When you are unfit your heart has to work harder and pump more times per minute to oxygenate the muscles. This puts a strain on the heart and makes it vulnerable to disease. With regular exercise you can enjoy a fitter, more active life, both now and as you age. This is particularly important today since the average life expectancy is rising.

For some people, incorporating regular exercise into their present lifestyle may seem impossible; but it really is not. The secret is to find a form of exercise which you enjoy. An easy solution is to use fitness equipment in the home. The most popular of these machines is the exercise bicycle. This a particularly effective form of exercise as it minimises the weight on the leg joints and is excellent for all age groups. Rowing and jogging are other popular outdoor sports which can be brought indoors with the use of machines.

If you have not exercised for a long time or are over 30, it is important that you begin exercising gently. If you attempt exercise which is too strenuous, the heart may be dangerously strained. It is always advisable to consult your doctor before you begin an exercise programme. Whereas younger or fitter people would have no difficulties in participating in active pursuits such as football, dancing or running, older people can find greater benefit from gentle forms of exercise such as cycling, golf or walking.

In addition to a healthier heart and a consequently reduced risk of heart disease, regular exercise can bring improvements in your general health. People who have taken up regular exercise after a long period of not exercising find they have more energy and vitality, and sleep better at night.

It is not too late to start exercising even if you have already suffered a heart attack. Healthcare professionals recommend gentle exercise to gradually restrengthen the heart muscle and to reduce the risk of further attacks.

2

ORTHODOX MEDICINE: WHAT CAN YOUR GP OFFER?

Having a healthy heart is central to your quality of life and achieving good heart health depends very largely on your lifestyle. The type of heart disease you are most likely to be familiar with is the sort that causes heart attacks. This is called *ischaemic heart disease,* or *coronary heart disease,* because it involves narrowing of the coronary arteries which supply blood to the heart. Britain today has an increasing number of people suffering from this condition and, unlike the USA and Australia, the incidence does not seem to be falling. It is frighteningly common, killing one man in five before the age of 65 and one woman in seven in the same age group.

Your family doctor is in a good position to advise you on ways of reducing your chances of a heart attack and to put information into some kind of perspective. There are many factors which can contribute to the risk and *your* risk will be different from anyone else's. Questions often come to mind when a relative or friend is taken ill with angina or a heart attack and suddenly everyone becomes aware that it could, in time, happen to them. It is a pity that it is only through fear that many people seek advice and information. Seeing your doctor provides the opportunity for examination and investigation, if appropriate.

Nearly every surgery now has a practice nurse who is able to do basic screening of patients for heart disease. This will include taking a family history, talking about diet, exercise, smoking and drinking habits, and even counselling about stress reduction. A cholesterol check, in the form of a blood test, may be offered. Some health visitors may also be involved in lifestyle counselling for the whole family.

The following pages describe the main factors contributing to heart disease and advice is given on how you can avoid them. There is still a lot for medical science to discover, even though technology has made treatment of heart problems safer and more successful.

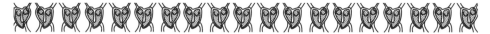

Ischaemic Heart Disease

When coronary heart disease occurs the arteries surrounding the heart become furred up and narrowed by fatty material known as atheroma (see page 19). These arteries are then unable to supply the heart muscle with enough oxygen for it to function properly. The result is angina, or, if the blood supply is totally cut off to one part of the heart, a myocardial infarction, commonly known as a heart attack. Preventing the arteries from developing fatty deposits and keeping the heart muscle fit are the fundamental aims of heart health.

For those of you who already have heart problems, there is still a lot that can be done. There is increasing evidence from research that changing habits, such as diet and smoking, can bring about a decrease in the amount of fatty deposits in coronary arteries and reduce the risk of another heart attack. The three main risk factors are cholesterol, smoking and hypertension. When more than one of these factors is present, their effect is multiplied and other factors, such as obesity and diabetes, may also compound the risk.

Cholesterol

This is the fatty substance found in fatty foods of animal origin (see page 41). A great deal of research has been conducted on how and why levels of this substance vary between different nationalities and within certain populations. These studies have shown a strong and direct link between the level of cholesterol in the blood and the incidence of coronary heart disease (CHD). However, cholesterol levels must always be considered in the light of other factors such as smoking; drastically reducing your cholesterol but continuing to smoke 40 cigarettes a day will do little to decrease your risk of a heart attack!

You may have a cholesterol blood test taken for a variety of reasons, especially if you are overweight, have any of the risk factors or if a close relative has died at an early age, say under 50, from a heart attack. Blood will be sent to the local hospital for analysis but your doctor may have a machine in the surgery which measures cholesterol with just a single drop of blood, the results being available in a few minutes. Levels are measured in *millimoles per litre* (*mmol/l*) and for Britain the desirable upper limit is 5.2 mmol/l. This really means that above this level your risk of a heart attack or

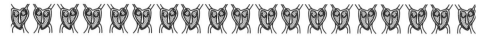

angina starts to increase considerably. Unfortunately, it does not mean that below that level you are immune to one! Levels above this should be monitored and you will be given appropriate advice about diet. There are several medical conditions which can raise cholesterol levels, for example, an underactive thyroid gland and diabetes, and these should be checked if your level is elevated. If, despite all this, the level remains raised above 7.5 mmol/l then your GP may consider starting you on treatment with a *lipid fat lowering agent*, which is described on page 30.

Some people are found to have extremely high levels indeed and many of these will be found to have the condition *familial hyperlipidaemia.*This is caused by a genetic abnormality affecting the liver. It can cause very premature heart disease and usually means that the whole family should be screened, even children. Anyone with a high cholesterol level in the range of 11.0 mmol/l and above really needs referral to a specialist to exclude this condition.

There is another type of fat in the blood called *triglyceride* which can be measured in the same way as cholesterol. In some studies it has been linked strongly to CHD but in others the link is less conclusive than that of cholesterol. Nonetheless, high levels of triglyceride in the blood should be lowered, starting with dietary measures (see Chapter 3).

Dietary Guidelines

Losing weight is the major goal as this will reduce cholesterol levels in most people automatically and the risk for CHD goes down. However, not all people with high cholesterol levels are overweight and more specific advice is then needed. Your GP will give you guidelines and there may be a dietician attached to the practice or at the local hospital if there are particular additional problems, such as diabetes. There is also a good deal of literature available at your doctor's practice and at the public library, and there is a large number of books on nutrition and special diets which provide low-fat recipes. In general, you will be advised to cut down on all red meats and dairy products which are high in saturated fat. The protein content of a healthy, low-cholesterol diet should be moderate amounts of white meat, such as chicken and fish, and plenty of pulses and lentils. It is amazing how difficult it is to encourage people to change their habits and to move the focus of a meal away from meat towards a variety of fish or vegetarian dishes but the effort is worth it.

There is now good evidence that particular sorts of fish are beneficial and reduce coronary heart disease. These are the fatty fish, such as mackerel, salmon and herring, which contain *polyunsaturated fats.* Olive oil and similar oils which contain *monounsaturates* are thought to have a preventive role in CHD as well but it is unclear why this is so. The other important factor is fibre. The average British diet contains approximately 20 gm of fibre daily and this should be increased to 30 gm ideally. It is easy to do this with the introduction of wholemeal bread and whole grain cereals. Dried fruit, nuts and pulses are all useful sources of fibre, too. The main theme should be variety and experimentation so that you are able to find foods that you like. There is no need to add bran to everything if you alter the rest of your diet appropriately.

Garlic is thought to be beneficial, too. Studies of people taking a clove of garlic per day showed that there was a decrease in cholesterol levels of 15 per cent. Garlic also has the ability to thin the blood and stop it from clotting inappropriately. Its exact mode of action is not known but it may account for the lower incidence of CHD in southern Europeans.

After starting a cholesterol-lowering and weight-reducing diet, a minimum of three months, sometimes six, is needed to see if the cholesterol level has fallen. Repeat levels should be taken after fasting overnight for at least 12 hours. If the levels are still high at this time, that is, over 8.0 mmol/l, treatment with a lipid lowering agent may be necessary. Most GPs will prescribe the drugs themselves but if you have other problems or take other medication then referral to a specialist clinic may be appropriate.

Lipid lowering agents.

- *Anion exchange resins,* for example, *cholestyramine* (trade name: Questran) were among the first drugs to be marketed for lowering blood fats. They are given as granules and can be quite unpalatable to take. While they are often effective, they are not free of side-effects and can cause *nausea* (the feeling of sickness) and abdominal discomfort. They can interfere with the absorption of some other drugs and also some vitamins, so they need to be taken under medical supervision, especially when given to children, but they are relatively safe.
- The *clofibrate* group of drugs includes *bezafibrate* (trade name: Bezalip) and *gemfibrizol* (trade name: Lopid) The main action of these is to decrease triglyceride levels but they also affect cholesterol to some

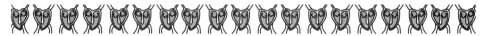

extent. They are generally more pleasant to take as they come in capsule form but they can still cause indigestion and nausea as well as rashes.

- The nicotinic acid group includes *nicotinic acid* and *nicofuranose* (trade name: Bradilan). The dose of these tablets needs to be increased gradually to minimise side-effects. They can cause flushing, rashes and dizziness in some people and are used less often than the other drugs.
- *Omega-3 marine triglycerides* is a prescribable form of fish oil for those who are unable or unwilling to tolerate eating sufficient fatty fish to lower their triglyceride levels. It is a well-tolerated medicine but occasionally causes nausea.
- *Statins* are drugs that block the manufacture of cholesterol by the body. They are the latest generation of drugs and are the most potent.

Hypertension

High blood pressure is also linked strongly with CHD and its discovery and treatment are matters handled largely by the family doctor or in conjunction with the practice nurse. Everyone should have a blood pressure check at three yearly intervals and this check will be offered routinely if you are changing doctors for any reason as part of a new patient registration check up. It is important to realise that having raised blood pressure may not cause you any symptoms at all unless the level is extremely high. It is measured in two parts, typically 130/80. The upper figure relates to the pressure, in millimetres of mercury, that is in the main blood vessels when the heart contracts. The lower figure is the pressure when the heart is relaxed. These are known as *systolic* and *diastolic* pressures respectively. Research has shown that a raised diastolic pressure increases risk for CHD and stroke more than systolic pressure, but both should be taken into account when considering treatment.

Blood pressure rises with age but studies clearly show that even mild hypertension should be treated and that it benefits people over 65 as well. Reduced incidence of stroke is more marked in this age group than reduced incidence of heart attacks.

There are many factors which can contribute to raised blood pressure but most people develop it for reasons as yet unknown. It is then called *essential hypertension*. There is a strong familial tendency to this so it is always worth getting your blood pressure checked if a close relative develops hypertension.

High blood pressure is commoner in people who smoke and who are overweight. Staying fit and active has been shown to have a protective effect as well as various forms of relaxation including meditation. The blood pressure level needs to be checked several times over a period of several months before considering treatment. Up to half of all people observed in this way will have blood pressures which fall to normal levels in this time without treatment. It is not entirely clear why this happens, but it may be related to the amount of anxiety generated when blood pressure is taken, which becomes less as the person becomes used to the procedure. Your doctor will decide if and when treatment is necessary. The most common treatments are *diuretics* (drugs that increase the flow of urine), for example, *bendrofluazide,* and *beta blockers* (drugs that decrease the activity of the heart), for example, *atenolol* (trade name: Tenormin). There is available a group of drugs which work on the kidneys, called *ACE* (*angiotensin converting enzyme*) *inhibitors,* such as *captopril.*

Once treatment is started it should be continued for life. Only about 10 per cent of people continue to have normal blood pressure when treatment is discontinued; the rest need to restart it. However, the benefits are proven and most people remain free of side-effects from the medication and are able to live a normal life.

Smoking

Only a third of the population of this country now smokes but it is still the major factor involved in deaths from heart disease. As described earlier, if you smoke and have another risk factor, such as being overweight, the risk of a heart attack is compounded. More than half of smokers, when asked, say they want to stop but it is often not the risk of heart and lung disease that is the main motivating factor. A pregnancy or young children in the home, even the amount of money saved, seem to be more influential. One of the commonest excuses for not stopping is that it is too late. This is not entirely true because studies have shown the risk of heart attack and angina decrease almost immediately for smokers who stop. This reduction in risk continues for several years though it is never as low as for people who have never smoked. Risk of CHD is proportional to the number of cigarettes smoked per day and the number of years smoking.

If you visit the surgery to ask your doctor's advice several options may be available. Information about your personal risk of a heart attack should be given with the offer of support from your doctor or the practice nurse. Some practices offer relaxation classes or a stop

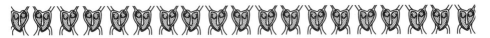

smoking support group. It is now possible to buy nicotine chewing gum and patches without a prescription.

Nicorette Gum

Available in 2 mg and 4 mg pieces, this was the first preparation on the market and it is still popular because it is placed in the mouth, like a cigarette. Nicotine from the gum takes a minute or two to have effect, rather longer than a drag on a cigarette, but each piece of gum lasts up to half an hour. The maximum recommended dose is fifteen 4 mg pieces in 24 hours. Some people get a sore mouth or ulcers with it but this is unusual. Usually after two or three months, the person will wean themselves off the gum. In rare cases there is some difficulty doing this and it may then be wise to change to the nicotine patches as described below. People experiencing difficulty might be offered counselling in the practice or with a psychologist.

Nicabate/Nicorette/Nicotinelle TTS Patches

Made by different pharmaceutical companies, these patches have a pouch which contains the nicotine in solution. The side which goes next to the skin is made of a membrane which allows slow release of the drug, which is absorbed through the skin at a constant rate and means that levels of nicotine in the blood remain fairly constant, avoiding withdrawal symptoms. Nicorette patches are used for 16 hours at a time and removed at night, while the other two preparations last 24 hours each and are used continuously. Each preparation has three different strengths, for example, Nicotinelle TTS comes in 15, 10 and 5 mg doses. The highest strength is used first and is replaced after three to six weeks with the next highest dose and so on until withdrawal is complete. Treatment is for three months in total with a review by the doctor recommended if withdrawal from them is not complete by then.

Alcohol

Excessive alcohol intake can damage almost any organ in the body, including the heart, directly. An intake of more than 14 units weekly (a unit is one pub measure of spirits, a glass of wine or half a pint of ordinary beer) is likely to cause a rise in cholesterol. Some people are reluctant to admit how much they drink to their GP and careful open questions are often needed to elicit the truth. (Moderate alcohol consumption is, however, strongly protective against heart disease in middle-aged and elderly men.)

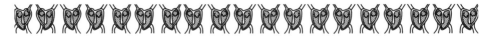

The type of treatment which a person with a drink problem will receive depends entirely on what they are prepared to accept. It is often the case that words of warning from family and friends are ignored but the doctor's advice is taken more seriously, especially when given in a clear and non-judgemental manner. Too often, though, some people continue to deny there is a problem, even when faced with evidence from a blood test or serious illness, that physical harm is being done.

Studies of problem drinkers have shown that success in stopping is much more likely if the person has a supportive spouse; a large part of help the GP will give is in providing support and guidance for family members. This includes referral to an appropriate agency, for example, Alcoholics Anonymous.

Diabetes

This relatively common illness is associated with increased cholesterol levels and an increased risk of CHD. The pancreas usually produces the hormone insulin in response to sugar levels in the blood and it enables the sugar to enter cells in the body to be used as energy. When the pancreas fails to produce enough insulin, levels of sugar rise and cause a variety of symptoms including excessive thirst, excessive amounts of urine and weight loss. When the condition is treated sufficiently, either with dietary measures, tablets or injectable insulin, the sugar levels drop and, following this, cholesterol levels will usually fall.

If you suffer from the above symptoms or if there is a family history of diabetes you should have a sample of urine tested for sugar.

Hypothyroidism

This occurs when the thyroid gland does not produce sufficient hormone to regulate the body's metabolic rate and the amount of fat in the bloodstream rises as a result. There is lethargy and weight gain in the person, who develops a husky voice and puffy facial features. This may be a familial condition and can be checked with a blood test. A lifetime of tablet treatment is then needed to replace the missing hormone which will usually correct the cholesterol level.

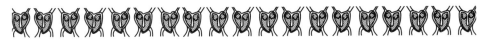

What if you already have heart disease?

It may be the case that you or one of your family already have heart disease. If this is so, it is helpful to go through some of the investigations and treatments that may be offered to help symptoms and to prevent further angina or heart attacks. Chest pain may be due to a large number of things and it is always wise to consult a doctor if you have recurrent pains, especially if this occurs on exercise or when you are feeling stressed.

An examination following a look at your full history may be all that is necessary for your GP to advise you of your risk for heart disease and how your lifestyle needs to change. If there is any doubt that you have angina, then a trial treatment is sometimes given even before any tests are done. This is usually in the form of *glyceryl trinitrate* as a tablet or spray under the tongue (see below). The commonest investigation is an ECG. This is usually done at the surgery and gives some idea of the size and shape of the heart, whether it is beating regularly and sometimes whether it is under strain. Looking at the heart at rest, however, may not give sufficient information so it is then necessary to repeat the test during exercise, for example, while walking on a treadmill. This may reveal heart strain that a resting ECG would miss.

If there is evidence of strain or damage, further tests will be performed which may include *coronary angiography*. A thin, flexible catheter is passed into a main blood vessel and into the entrance to the arteries round the heart. Dye is injected to highlight the blood vessels on X-ray and will show up any narrowing of coronary vessels. A decision to operate on these arteries may then be made so that the blood supply can be improved. This can be done in some people using a specially adapted *catheter* (a long, slender flexible tube) which widens the inside of the arteries. Otherwise a heart operation may be offered to bypass any blockage in the blood vessels round the heart. This is known as a *coronary artery bypass graft*. All these procedures are aimed at preventing or minimising further damage to heart muscle to keep it functioning effectively.

Drug Treatment

There are many drugs used to relieve and prevent the pain of angina. Some of these have been shown to provide protection against heart attacks and some act only on the symptoms. Below is a brief description of some of the drugs which have a protective effect

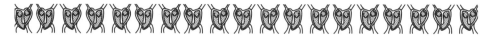

on the heart and those which are thought to minimise damage after a heart attack.

Beta Blockers

These drugs, for example, *atenolol* (trade name: Tenormin) and *propranolol* (trade name: Inderal), are used for a variety of conditions including high blood pressure and angina. They are also effective for anxiety and tension headaches to some extent. They act on the circulatory system by damping down the 'fight or flight' mechanism that is usually triggered by adrenaline. This slows the pulse rate and reduces blood pressure. They also have the effect of slightly constricting the airways to the lungs. This does not affect most people but can cause asthmatics to wheeze more and become more short of breath and so beta blockers need to be used with caution.

Beta blockers are given in tablet form although liquid is available. They can cause a variety of side-effects but are mostly well tolerated. Some people feel tired on them, or have nightmares, and a change to a slightly different formula can sometimes help.

Aspirin

You may be surprised to find this well-known over-the-counter drug included here but it has been shown in clinical trials that an aspirin tablet can reduce death from heart attacks if given within a short time of the attack. Aspirin acts on blood cells called *platelets* to make them less sticky. It is then less likely that the clot of blood in the coronary artery will extend. There is beneficial effect from continuing aspirin on a lifelong basis. This consists of just half an adult aspirin tablet daily or less (75 mg twice weekly is sufficient), and is the same treatment as given to people who have had a stroke. This dose of aspirin is unlikely to cause any indigestion.

Streptokinase Group Of Drugs

Routine use of these life-saving drugs is relatively new and is reserved for people who have had a definite heart attack within the previous 12 hours, it is best if they can be given within two hours of the heart attack. They are given directly into a vein, nearly always in hospital. They act on the clotting mechanism of the blood to dissolve rapidly any clot. They are also used for dissolving clots in the lungs and the leg. Their use may be dangerous if the person has had a previous stroke but it has been shown to be life saving when given appropriately. Following the injection, aspirin is given by mouth for at least the following four weeks.

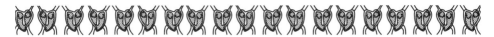

Other Types Of Heart Disease

There are several other types of heart disease that involve structures other than the coronary arteries although they are all less common than ischaemic heart disease.

Congenital Heart Disease

This is any disorder of the structure of the heart which is present from birth. One of the commonest defects is a hole between the upper or lower chambers of the heart. It is not always possible to find a cause for this. Quite a high proportion of these holes in the heart, known to doctors as *atrial septal* or *ventricular septal defects*, are small and will close up by themselves within a year of birth, making treatment unnecessary. They occur more commonly with conditions such as *Down's syndrome* and other chromosome disorders. Certain infections in the mother during the early weeks of pregnancy can also give rise to holes in the heart and other more complex defects. The best-known infection is *rubella* (also known as *German measles*). If this is contracted between 6 and 12 weeks of pregnancy, it is highly likely to cause damage to the heart and may damage other organs of the foetus as well. Immunity to rubella is routinely checked during early pregnancy, but any pregnant woman who thinks she has been in contact with the disease should seek medical advice urgently.

It is now routine to immunise teenage girls against rubella and this has helped to reduce its incidence considerably. Immunity can then be checked at a later date with a blood test. This test is available to all teenage girls and women of childbearing age. If you are planning a pregnancy, it is well worth having this test done first. If you are not immune to rubella, the immunisation can then be given and you must avoid pregnancy for three months afterwards.

Some forms of congenital heart disease can be inherited, although the reasons for this are not clear. Parents who have had one or more children with significant heart problems will be offered *genetic counselling* (the procedure by which patients and their families are given advice about the nature and consequences of inherited disorders) by a specialist if they are considering further pregnancies. Detailed *ultrasonic scans* (scans using sound waves) may be offered to the mother during subsequent pregnancies to check that the baby's heart is developing normally.

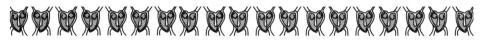

Palpitations

Nearly everyone experiences palpitations of some kind during their lives and they can be very worrying. Usually, though, this does not mean there is any heart disease present, especially in the absence of chest pain. Being tired or stressed, and drinking too much tea or coffee, can all precipitate awareness of the heart beating.

It is important to distinguish whether the palpitations are regular or irregular and how long they last. Below are some of the types of palpitation. Several do not require any action other than reassurance and a change in lifestyle.

Awareness of the heart missing a beat is common and due to *ectopic* (extra) beats from the upper or lower chamber of the heart. It does not indicate CHD and will tend to disappear on exercise. The heartbeat may just be felt as prominent though regular and this also is common and of no great significance. An irregular fast heartbeat could indicate the condition *atrial fibrillation*. This means that the upper chambers of the heart, *the atria*, are beating in an unco-ordinating fashion. This is a spontaneous occurrence in the elderly but in younger people should always be investigated as there may be an underlying physical illness or heart condition. Tablet treatment, such as with one of the anti-arrhythmic tablets, can help the heart rate to become slightly slower and some people spontaneously revert to normal rhythm in any case after a time.

Very fast, sustained heartbeat can be a warning sign of serious heart problems and medical advice should always be sought if it does not settle within a few minutes.

Bacterial Endocarditis

This is a rare but very serious condition which occurs in people who already have damage to their heart valves or congenital heart disease of some sort. It is an infection of the heart whereby bacteria settle and grow on the abnormal areas, causing the valves to become misshapen and to leak. The heart is unable to function properly and bacteria and debris may circulate in the blood, causing generalised illness or *septicaemia* (blood poisoning). Tiny *haemorrhages* (bleeding from ruptured vessels) in the fingers or feet may be one of the first signs of this. It is rare in people who have a completely normal heart. Admission to hospital is necessary and treatment is given in the form of antibiotics through a drip. All procedures, such as dental treatment and operations on the bladder or bowel, can

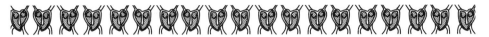

cause bacteria to enter the general circulation so preventive treatment in the form of antibiotics by mouth should be given to anyone who has a significant heart defect. (This does not usually mean people with coronary artery disease.) Anyone who has a heart *murmur* (a soft, abnormal sound) should seek medical advice and find out whether or not it is necessary for them to have antibiotics *prophylactically* (taken to prevent or protect against illness).

Rheumatic Fever

This potentially serious illness is now quite rare in Britain but was once relatively common when housing conditions and nutrition were less good. It is a *febrile* (feverish) illness caused by the bacterium *streptococcus.* This affects the heart valves and causes them to become misshapen. After some years, the heart valves cease to function properly, becoming too stiff to open and close properly, with the result that the heart begins to fail. Many older people who have had valve replacements had rheumatic fever in childhood. Improvements in social conditions and, to a lesser extent, antibiotics, have helped to prevent the illness almost completely in the 1990s.

Cardiomyopathy

A relatively rare condition, this occurs when the heart muscle becomes diseased. There is often no obvious reason for this. The heart muscle may overgrow and one of the symptoms of this is angina, due to inadequate blood supply to the extra muscle. Alternatively, the heart chambers may become dilated, making the pump mechanism inadequate. It is unclear why this happens, but it can occur with excessive alcohol intake. The heart is unable to pump blood adequately and heart failure develops with fluid in the lungs and ankle swelling. The outlook for this condition is fairly poor and it is one of the indications for a heart transplant in some cases.

Surgery

Operations on the heart have been performed on many thousands of patients in the last thirty years and, whatever the reason for the surgery, the chances of success are now higher than ever. There are many different operations which can be performed, depending on

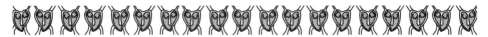

the age of the person and the exact physical problem with the heart.

The commonest operation is a coronary artery bypass graft which is mentioned earlier in the chapter and which involves cutting into the chest and exposing the heart; that is, open heart surgery. The portion of the diseased artery round the heart is bypassed using a vein which is removed from one of the legs. Alternatively, part of an artery from inside the chest wall may be used. This operation is the most usual in the UK although some operations are performed to widen the inside of coronary arteries using a catheter, as described above. There is some suggestion from studies that the long-term results from this treatment are less good than with open heart surgery but it is more suitable for people who are too ill to tolerate major surgery or who have a very small area of blocked artery. Catheter operations in the USA are much more common. The overall outcome is successful in 95 per cent of cases after one year.

Surgery to replace diseased heart valves is also now a common procedure, although the need for this is declining, along with the major reduction in the incidence of rheumatic fever. Occasionally it is possible to use the catheter method to widen a diseased valve, but this will not always restore it to normal function and is not a common operation. Two main types of replacement valve now exist, one in the shape of a disc and the other in the shape of a ball. When the valve is in place and the person has recovered, it is usually possible to hear the valve clicking inside the chest as it works. Everyone with a replacement heart valve needs lifetime treatment with tablets to thin the blood; usually the drug warfarin is used.

Heart transplant is the operation which over the years has attracted the most publicity but it is only a small minority of the total heart operations performed. Results in the short and medium term have improved as each year goes by but longer-term difficulties, with the person's immune system rejecting the transplant, still pose a problem, as they do with the transplant of other organs; the development of new drugs to prevent this rejection is now the most important advance needed.

Operations for severe congenital heart disease are a very specialised part of heart surgery and can carry high risk if the child is new-born and unwell. Such surgery is carried out in only a few centres in the UK. Less major surgery, however, such as repair of holes in the heart, has a very high success rate indeed, with almost no long-term effects on the child; in many children the operation is delayed until they are of an age and size to make anaesthesia a safe undertaking.

3

NUTRITION: EAT YOUR WAY TO A HEALTHY HEART

The Fats Of Life And Death

Not all fats are unhealthy. There are two types of fats: structural and storage. Storage fats, of which cholesterol is one, are predominantly saturated fats. They provide a long-term supply of energy to the body in times of food or energy shortage. Dietary surveys clearly demonstrate that we consume far too much cholesterol and other saturated fats, most of which are unnecessary because our bodies can and do manufacture both cholesterol and saturated fats from other sources.

It is now firmly established that excessive fat in the diet results in high blood cholesterol levels which in turn increase the risk of a heart attack. This is because cholesterol accumulates on the walls of the arteries to produce atherosclerosis (see page 19). In atherosclerosis blood platelets tend to collect, forming a clot around damaged areas, thus narrowing the artery and eventually blocking the blood supply, causing a heart attack.

On the other hand, structural fats, found in plants, vegetables and some fish, cannot be made by the body yet are vital for continued good health; for this reason they are known as *essential fats*. If these essential fats are lacking or not present in sufficient amounts in our food, they can have an undesirable effect on, among other things, cardiovascular health. Modern eating habits, farming methods and food processing contribute to a diet typically lacking in essential fats.

Role Of Cholesterol

Because cholesterol receives such a bad press its importance for our overall health is not usually appreciated. In fact, every cell in the body contains cholesterol. This fatty substance resides in our cell walls, where it helps to maintain the rigid structure of the cells. A properly intact cell wall is necessary to protect the delicate cell contents and so cholesterol's structural role is vital. Cholesterol is

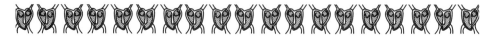

also needed for the formation of *bile salts* (which aid in the breakdown and absorption of fats) and is vital in the body for the production of steroid hormones. It is the raw material from which the sex and adrenal hormones are made.

A Matter Of Balance

Cholesterol is manufactured in the liver. Like other fats, cholesterol is not soluble in water and is therefore insoluble in blood *plasma* (the fluid portion of blood in which the cells etc. are suspended). As such, cholesterol is transported in the body in the form of compounds known as *lipoproteins.* Lipoproteins are small droplets with a central core of cholesterol, tryglycerides and other fats surrounded by an outer shell of water-soluble protein molecules. The percentage of proteins these droplets contain determines their density and size. The small, heavy and highly compressed ones are called *high density lipoproteins* (*HDL*) and the larger and loosely packed ones are called *low density lipoproteins* (*LDL*).

The main role of LDL is to transport cholesterol from the liver to parts of the body where it is needed. HDL carries unwanted cholesterol back to the liver, but its primary function is to scavenge excess cholesterol which is left in potentially health-damaging places, such as the artery walls. Problems arise when there is a shortage of HDL to eliminate accumulated cholesterol.

Triglycerides: Unwanted Body Fat

Besides cholesterol, there is another dietary substance which increases the risk of heart disease: triglycerides. Indeed, some experts believe that triglyceride levels are an even more important indicator of cardiovascular risk than cholesterol. An increased level of triglycerides make the blood more viscous and more likely to produce clots which might lodge in a narrowed artery. Triglyceride fats are an important energy source, richer in energy than sugar or carbohydrate. The fats you see on top of a bottle of full cream milk or the lardy part of meat and plant fats (oils) are triglycerides.

Fats Explained

There are three common types of fats: saturated, polyunsaturated and monounsaturated.

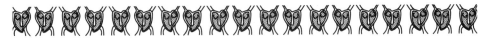

The type of fat in our diet bears major implications on our health, in particular our heart health. The differences between the types of fats lie in their chemistry, specifically the way in which the carbon and hydrogen atoms are linked. All fats contain carbon and hydrogen atoms. A single link between the carbon atoms describes a saturated fat, a double link an unsaturated fat. A monounsaturated fat has one double link, while a polyunsaturated fat has two or more double links. Translating the chemistry into actual foods, lard (hard fat), for example, is composed mainly of saturated fats while olive oil is mainly composed of monounsaturated fats. Corn and vegetable oils are mostly polyunsaturated fats.

Saturated fats raise cholesterol levels while dietary polyunsaturated fats lower them. But which fats increase or decrease the level of 'bad' LDL cholesterol, and maintain the level of 'good' HDL cholesterol?

Fish oils have been found to be most beneficial for heart health. The active substance in fish oils is *omega-3*, a name which sounds as though it belongs in the realms of science fiction rather than nutrition. The effects of omega-3 are very real, however: it affects total blood cholesterol, LDL, with simultaneous boosting of HDL. Omega-3 is one of a group of *essential fatty acids* (*EFAs*) primarily found in oily fish, such as mackerel, salmon and herring.

Fatty fish, such as salmon, can therefore reduce the risk of heart disease because their oil is rich in omega-3. Fish oil is the oil which is squeezed from the muscle of oily fish. This is different from cod liver oil which is squeezed from the liver rather than the flesh. Cod liver oil is rich in vitamins A and D but does not necessarily have as much essential fatty acid content as fish oil.

The vital ingredients in fish oil are two tongue-twisting fatty acids: *eicosapentaenoic acid* (*EPA*) and *docosahexaenoic acid* (*DHA*). These essential fatty acids are required by both fish and humans. However, neither humans nor fish can manufacture these themselves and rely on obtaining them from food.

Eskimos And Fish Oils

Dr Hugh Sinclair, a nutritional biochemist, was the first to identify the bizarre conundrum of the Eskimos: despite their diet, one which includes the highest animal fat content in the world, their blood cholesterol levels are exceptionally low. Of interest to Western

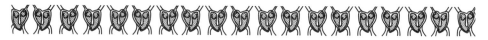

scientists was the remarkably low incidence of both heart disease and rheumatoid arthritis among the Eskimo population. Could the West learn something of interest from the Eskimos?

Dr Sinclair journeyed to Greenland in 1976, accompanied by two Danish scientists, John Dyerberg and Hans Bang, to further study the Eskimo phenomenon. Analysis of the fats in the Eskimo's blood showed high levels of the omega-3 essential fatty acids. Eskimos consume some 2 $^1/_2$ lb of fatty fish each day (an intake of 6 g of omega-3 acids). The old wives' tale that fish is good for you was therefore found to be scientifically accurate because of the presence of omega-3 in fish oils.

Fish Oils And Health

A number of studies have been carried out which graphically illustrate the effects of fish oils not only on heart health but also on arthritis, foetal development and several skin conditions.

A 20-year study in the Netherlands (1960–1980), which involved middle-aged men without a history of coronary heart disease, demonstrated that those who consumed at least 1.1 oz of fish a day had only half the death rate from heart attacks as those who did not eat fish.

In Wales in 1983, a study was set up by the Medical Research Council to determine whether men who had already suffered a heart attack could reduce the risk of further attacks by a change in their diets. The results demonstrated that the group of men which had increased their consumption of fatty fish had 29 per cent fewer deaths than the group which had not.

Two thousand men, who had already had a heart attack and were therefore at a higher than normal risk of an attack, were randomly divided into three groups and each group was given different dietary advice. The first group was advised to cut down on total fat intake. The second group was put on a high-fibre cereal diet and the men in the third group were asked to eat oil-rich fish. Those who could not, or would not, eat fish were offered fish oil capsules. The men were monitored for a period of two years and researchers found that a third fewer men died of heart attack in the fish group compared to each of the other two groups.

Today we eat far less fish than previous generations, in particular fatty fish, such as mackerel and herrings, which are the primary dietary source of omega-3 essential fatty acids. Yet the evidence

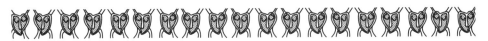

suggests that adding fish oil to the diet does a lot of good. All you need to do is to take one or two portions of oily fish a week and two or three fish oil capsules a day to ensure that you have sufficient amounts of omega-3 (about 1 g).

Fish Rich In Omega-3 Polyunsaturates

- Mackerel
- Herrings
- Sardines
- Tuna (fresh)
- Lake trout
- Salmon

Effects of Omega-3 Polyunsaturates

- Reduce the risk of heart disease
- Reduce the likelihood of blood clot formation
- Make the blood less viscous
- Improve the immune function and other body systems

How Much Cholesterol Is Too Much?

The answer to this question has to take into account the fact that our bodies do not actually need a dietary source of cholesterol at all. The liver manufactures cholesterol and, quite simply, can make sufficient amounts with no need for further dietary sources.

Estimates suggest that, to minimise health risks, the amount of cholesterol in the diet should be no more than 200–300 mg per day. This is only a small allowance – the equivalent of an egg.

Some Cholesterol-Rich Foods

- Brains 1480 mg/100 g
- Kidney 804 mg/100 g
- Whole egg 504 mg/100 g
- Liver 438 mg
- Heart (beef) 274 mg/100 g
- Double cream 133 mg/100 g

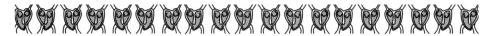

The Fibre Connection

Dietary fibre (from fruits, vegetables, grains and seeds) has an active effect against cholesterol. This is because fibre tends to bind with cholesterol in the gut and so prevents its reabsorption in the body. Fibre also encourages the growth of intestinal bacteria, which again is advantageous, as some of these bacteria degrade cholesterol into products which are very difficult for the body to absorb from the gut.

Plant foods also contain another component which is, quite literally, nature's 'cholesterol neutraliser'. The substance is *beta-sitosterol* and can be regarded as the plant equivalent of cholesterol. However, far from having the same harmful effects as cholesterol, beta-sitosterol actually blocks the absorption of cholesterol in the intestine. It does this by competing with cholesterol for the same absorption sites on the intestinal wall. The body 'mistakes' beta-sitosterol for cholesterol, tries to absorb it, finds that it cannot and therefore releases the beta-sitosterol again. Meanwhile cholesterol has passed through the body unabsorbed.

Vegetable oils, especially corn oil, are the best source of beta-sitosterol. Unfortunately, modern oilseed processing techniques remove much of this valuable substance from the final product.

Most of the blood cholesterol-lowering substances, such as garlic, fish oils, vitamin C, niacin, and lecithin, achieve their purpose by mobilising cholesterol so that it can be transported to the liver. But by virtue of the fact that cholesterol is converted in the liver to bile salts, much cholesterol actually ends up back in the intestine again. Here there is a danger that it will simply be reabsorbed. Therefore, although the above substances do have a well-documented value in reducing cholesterol levels, their efficiency is even further enhanced by the presence of beta-sitosterol in the diet at the same time.

Cholesterol alone does not cause heart attacks, but an elevated blood cholesterol is invariably present in a potential heart victim. By taking care to lower blood cholesterol, untold suffering can be avoided.

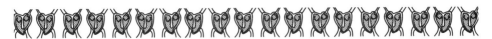

The Fats Of Life And Death

High Total Fat Intake

- Dietary fat is the most difficult food component to digest. Protein and carbohydrates in excess of energy needs are readily converted to fat for energy storage.
- A general indicator of health is one percentage of body fat compared to lean body mass. In general, leaner individuals, especially men, experience less disease of all types.

What This Means

- Fat calories in excess of the optimal amount will result in an overly full feeling (which some people crave) and body fat storage which has long-term health consequences.
- A high-density-calorie diet results in a comfortably full feeling. Modifying the calorie content of the diet can be difficult when going on a low-fat, high-fibre, high-nutrient-density diet to lose weight.
- Dietary fats convert more readily to body fat storage than either carbohydrates or protein. Habituation to the comfortable post-meal feeling of a high-fat diet may indicate poor blood sugar regulation, with dietary fat slowing down carbohydrate absorption.
- Obesity and clogging of arteries result from years of a high-fat diet.

How To Make Changes

- Learn about the fat content of separate food ingredients and the foods in which the ingredients appear. Select low-fat foods wherever a choice is available, for example, yogurts and salad dressings. Remove the skin from chicken and fat from meats. Order low-fat items, such as chicken and fish, when dining out, and ask for dressing and sour cream on the side.
- Food fats are found abundantly in animal source foods, such as eggs, meat, cheese, milk and sour cream. Generally, fat and protein characterise animal foods and fibre, carbohydrate and protein characterise plant foods.

Low Total Fat Intake

- The fat content of a meal will determine how fast the meal empties from the stomach. Very-low-fat diets are uncomfortable because one never feels full for very long; however, adjusting to a low-fat diet will be

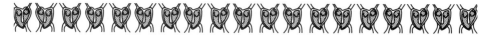

well worth the effort in health improvement.
- Low-fat diets correlate with a lower incidence of heart attacks.

What This Means

- Fat is found in almost every food and is used commonly in preparation methods.
- Eat low-fat foods more often to avoid the fat-satisfaction connection.
- A low-fat diet may also reduce the consumption of the fat-soluble vitamins, A, D and E. If nutrient-dense foods are selected, this should not be a problem.
- Food fats from fish and selected plant sources should be included for optimal health. Supplementation is indicated where dietary preferences do not permit this.

How To Make Changes

- Select foods with good fats, such as cold water fish, and reduce saturated fats from animal products.
- Fats are found abundantly in the food supply. Good fats are found in fish, olive oil and flaxseed oil.

High Monounsaturated Fat Intake

- Cultures using olive oil, famous for its high monounsaturated fatty acid content, are remarkably free of heart disease, even with high total fat calories.

What This Means

- Incorporating olive oil into cooking is an easy step in making total dietary changes. A diet low in monounsaturated fats will have no short-term effects, but if the total fat calories are high, health problems can be predicted.
- With total fat calories held at the optimal range, a greater percentage of monounsaturated fats will lower the LDL cholesterol and keep the HDL level constant.
- There are no studies indicating any correlation with high monounsaturated fat intake and health problems when total fat calories are in the optimum range. This is not so for saturated fats (which can cause heart disease) and polyunsaturated fats (which can be implicated in some types of cancer).

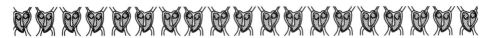

How To Make Changes

- Seek out recipes and styles of cooking that use olive oil as cooking fat. Use this sparingly to keep total fat calories as low as possible.

Low Monounsaturated Fat Intake

- Monounsaturated fats lower the bad LDL cholesterol while leaving good HDL cholesterol alone. Polyunsaturated fats lower both HDL and LDL cholesterol simultaneously and defeat the benefit of having a high HDL to LDL ratio.

What This Means

- The onset of heart disease can be delayed or possibly avoided by using monounsaturated oils in the diet. Heart disease may take decades to become apparent, but is a gradual ongoing process that requires dietary modification today for health rewards later in life.
- Underconsumption of the monounsaturated fats and the resultant overconsumption of polyunsaturated, unsaturated and saturated fats may predispose an individual to heart disease.
- The blood fat conditions that contribute to heart disease are produced by saturated fats. High total dietary fat will contribute to poor health, but a low fat intake, of primarily monounsaturated fats, will contribute to optimal health.

How To Make Changes

- Use olive oil for cooking in place of butter or margarine. Look for foods containing a high monounsaturated fat content (high *oleic acid*), and use olive oil in marinades, dressings, etc.
- Food sources include olive oil and flaxseed oil.

High Polyunsaturated Fat Intake

- Polyunsaturated fatty acids (PUFA) are generally thought to be healthier than saturated fats, but not as healthy as monounsaturated fats. Vegetable oils, such as sunflower and soya, are rich in PUFA.
- PUFA lower the total cholesterol, but do not achieve the desired effect of increasing the HDL to LDL ratio. Exercise and monounsaturated fats achieve this goal.

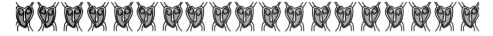

What This Means

- Too high PUFA in addition to high total fat will result in rapid weight gain.
- PUFA that are rancid contribute to immune suppression, heart disease and accelerated ageing. Fresh oils found in health food stores, purchased in small bottles for rapid use and stored in a cool, dark place, e.g. the fridge, will minimise the risks.

How To Make Changes

- Incorporate olive oil into cooking methods and add fish to your diet to achieve a balance between the good fats and the bad fats.
- Food sources of PUFA include corn, soya, sunflower and safflower oils.

Low Polyunsaturated Fat Intake

- PUFA are found mainly in plant sources. They tend to lower total cholesterol levels without favourably altering the important HDL to LDL cholesterol level.

What This Means

- Linoleic and linolenic PUFA are essential fatty acids required daily for optimal health. The amount of fat that supplies the daily amount is small: two pats of butter or margarine, or two teaspoons of vegetable oil.
- A low intake of PUFA may indicate over-consumption of animal fats, which are mostly saturated. A low overall fat intake is desirable, with a focus on monounsaturated fats. Skin problems, especially dry and itchy skin, may indicate a deficiency of PUFA.

How To Make Changes

- If saturated fats are being overconsumed at the expense of PUFA, select plant fat sources rather than animal sources, especially olive oil.
- The total fat intake in the diet should be as low as possible, but the ratio of saturated, mono-and polyunsaturated should be balanced.
- Food sources of PUFA include corn, soya, sunflower and safflower oils.

High Saturated Fat Intake

- Animal foods, such as dairy foods and red meat, are high in saturated fats. Conventional nutritional thinking targets high saturated fat consumption as a serious health risk leading to heart disease. A

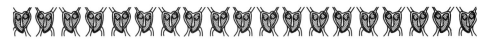

commitment to change and dietary modification will be necessary to correct a high saturated fat intake.

- High fat diets usually are low in fibre. Increasing fibre and antioxidant vitamins such as C and E and beta carotene can help offset some of the harm the fat presents.

What This Means

- A high saturated fat intake is common in Western cultures where animal foods are regularly consumed. The health effects may take several decades to become apparent.
- Heart disease is the long-term effect of a diet too high in saturated fats. Dietary habits and food preferences are learned in childhood and change requires constant effort and a strong commitment.
- Clogging of the arteries will result from the high triglyceride and cholesterol production stimulated by high saturated fats in the diet. The more saturated a fat is, the more solid it is at room temperature. This explains why saturated fats clog arteries rather than stay fluid in the blood.
- Heavy consumption of animal fats with their higher proportion of saturated fats will predispose an individual to heart disease. Only animal fats contain cholesterol, but all saturated fats can provoke higher cholesterol production by the liver. Palm and coconut oils are highly saturated plant fats and for this reason they are known health risks.

How To Make Changes

- Select fats from vegetable sources while keeping total fat intake as low as possible. Incorporate skinned chicken and fish as alternative protein sources to red meat.
- Animal foods contain mainly saturated fat and cholesterol in varying degrees. A switch to vegetable protein sources for part of the daily protein intake will increase fibre (highly desirable) and eliminate a source of cholesterol.
- Avoid saturated fats found in animal food sources such as meat, eggs, cheese and milk.

Low Saturated Fat Intake

- Saturated fats are found in animal foods in high levels.
- Saturated fats are desirable in some processed foods due to their solid

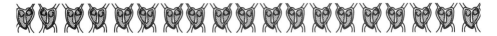

nature. For example, cocoa butter melts at human body temperature and gives chocolate its smooth properties.
- Saturated fats provoke an increase in cholesterol synthesis by the liver, so a reduction of saturated fats is necessary to lower cholesterol levels.

What This Means
- The human body can synthesise all fats except for linoleic and linolenic fatty acids. The absolute minimum amount of fat required in the diet can be found in two servings of butter or margarine or in two teaspoons of vegetable oil per day.

How To Make Changes
- Generally, the lowest fat diet that is tolerable is the healthiest. Monounsaturated fats from olive oil are healthier than either saturated or polyunsaturated fats.
- Saturated fats are found in animal food sources such as meat, eggs, cheese and milk.

Garlic

Wood and clay carvings of garlic have been found in the tombs of pharaohs. From this we can assume that the ancient Egyptians had discovered the health-giving properties of this herb and wanted to guarantee the health of the pharaohs' spirit in the afterlife. An Egyptian papyrus of around 1550 BC includes 22 therapeutic recipes which use garlic for complaints ranging from animal bites to heart problems and tumours. The Egyptians were not alone in their belief in the curative powers of garlic: the Greeks, Romans and Vikings have all left us evidence that garlic was prescribed both as a preventative measure against disease and as a cure for a variety of illnesses. And Louis Pasteur reported on garlic's anti-bacterial activity in 1858 when he used garlic as an antiseptic.

Today, garlic has seized the interest of research scientists around the world – so much so that the first World Congress on the Health Significance of Garlic and Garlic Constituents was held in 1990. Among the many papers presented at the Congress, one by Dr Robert Lin suggested that a daily dose of garlic and garlic extract can substantially reduce the risk of cancer and cardiovascular disease.

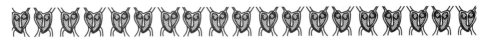

How Does Garlic Improve Cardiovascular Health?

We have seen that cardiovascular health is at risk as a result of high blood pressure, high cholesterol levels and high platelet stickiness. Garlic affects all three of these factors beneficially and consequently lessens the risk of heart disease, providing, of course, that a reasonably healthy lifestyle is maintained.

Garlic's Effect On Blood Pressure

Garlic appears to lower high blood pressure, perhaps by having a dilatory effect on the blood vessels and so reducing pressure. Whatever the (as yet unknown) reason, trials on 100 patients with abnormally high blood pressure showed a significant reduction in blood pressure in 40 people after just one week's dosage of garlic. Chinese herbalists have, in fact, used garlic to relieve high blood pressure for many years and it is a part of their standard practice.

Garlic's Effect On Cholesterol

In a Japanese study, garlic was tested for its effects on cholesterol. Thirty-two subjects with high levels of cholesterol were randomly divided into two groups. Members of the first group were given a liquid of aged garlic extract while members of the second group were given a *placebo* (an inactive substance). Blood levels were measured every month for a period of six months. In the first two months of the study those on aged garlic actually suffered an increase in cholesterol. In the third month the level started to drop, reaching normal at the end of six months. Researchers explained the initial rise in cholesterol as due to the ability of garlic to shift fats from the tissues where they have been accumulated back into the bloodstream.

Garlic's Effect On Platelets

We know that a heart attack occurs when a blood clot forms in one of the arteries leading to the heart. Blood clots are formed when platelets build up and become trapped with red blood cells in *fibrin*, which is a mesh-like substance. High cholesterol levels, smoking, stress and numerous other factors make the platelets stickier and consequently slow down blood flow. Garlic extract reduces platelet stickiness because it contains *ajoene*, an anticlotting factor.

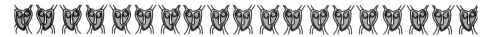

Aged Garlic

The aged garlic used in clinical trials is different from the garlic bulbs used in cooking. The pungent smell of garlic is only released when the cloves are cut or crushed; doing so releases the active ingredients – the amino acid *alliin* and and the enzyme *allinase*. The amino acid and the enzyme fuse to produce a new substance: *allicin*, and it is this which produces garlic's pungent odour.

Allicin is very unstable and oxidises at temperatures above 4°C into many sulphur-based compounds. It is this unique spectrum of sulphur-containing nutrients that lends garlic its health-giving properties.

Traditional Chinese herbalists use garlic cloves which have been aged for two to three years in vinegar for a variety of health complaints. Today, garlic is aged by slicing it (without using heat) and leaving it in stainless steel tanks for approximately 20 months. During this 'cold-ageing' time, as it is known, the alliin is converted via allicin to a whole host of new beneficial garlic compounds, so that cold-aged garlic is reputed to have more health benefits than ordinary garlic preparations. The end product of the cold-ageing process is odourless, making it socially acceptable. Cold-aged garlic is available both in liquid and tablet form.

Lecithin

Lecithin supplementation also appears to be effective in reducing blood cholesterol and has earned itself a reputation as a vital nutrient in the prevention and treatment of heart disease, since it is a natural *emulsifier*, i.e. it enables fats and water to mix.

Lecithin was first isolated in 1850. It is manufactured by the liver but is also found in egg yolk and in soya beans (it is this source which is widely used today). Lecithin is primarily fat combined with phosphorus. The ingredients active in controlling cholesterol and helping the metabolism to burn fat and turn it into energy are agents called *phospholipids*. These link with substances called *choline* and *inositol*.

Being a fat, cholesterol does not mix with water and, if left on its own, will not pass into the blood but instead will remain in the arteries where it will eventually build up deposits if it is not absorbed. As an emulsifier, lecithin can effect absorption of cholesterol into the rest of the body's cells, so avoiding harmful

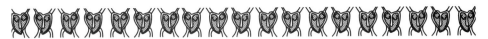

cholesterol deposits. Various studies of sufferers of coronary heart disease have shown low levels of blood lecithin, with a corresponding increased risk of blood clotting. Furthermore, stickiness of blood platelets is decreased by polyunsaturated fatty acids and linolenic acid: lecithin is rich in both. This in turn has an effect on levels of good and bad cholesterol – HDL and LDL respectively – by increasing levels of the former and decreasing the latter.

Vitamin C

Vitamin C plays a valuable role in numerous ways in protecting the arteries, not least of which is keeping the artery walls healthy. It aids in the reversal of plaque formation and mobilises arterial deposits of cholesterol. Not only does vitamin C affect the total cholesterol content of the blood but it also positively influences the HDL/LDL ratio and regulates triglyceride levels.

Vitamin C is perhaps the most researched antioxidant substance. It is soluble in water and provides antioxidant protection for the watery compartments of our cells, tissues and organs. Our bodies cannot manufacture vitamin C so we are dependent upon food sources for this vital nutrient.

Vitamin E

Alpha tocopherol, to give vitamin E its other name, is an important nutrient which, in common with vitamin C and beta carotene, plays a crucial role in heart health. It is thought to affect the balance of prostaglandins in favour of decreased blood clotting and blood platelets and hence its importance in heart health. In January 1991, the *Lancet* reported a study of relationships between vitamins C and E by a group of investigators in Switzerland and Scotland. They observed that the risk of developing angina is increased by nearly three times when there is a low plasma level of vitamins C and E. Furthermore, the relationship between low plasma levels of vitamin C and angina was found to be substantially influenced by smoking habits.

It is also thought that a low dietary intake of vitamins E and C may increase the chances of a *thrombosis* (blood clot in a blood vessel) and impedes the normal contraction of heart muscle.

Vitamin E has a very powerful antioxidant effect on the body,

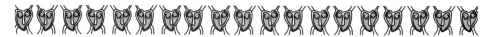

particularly protecting the lipids in cell walls (lipids are particularly susceptible to oxidation by free radicals). It also protects the oxidation of polyunsaturated fatty acids by free radicals.

Vitamin E is enhanced by other antioxidants, such as vitamin C and the mineral selenium. Quantities of vitamin E are expressed in either of two ways: by weight (mg) or as a biological activity (iu).

Foods rich in vitamin E include oils (wheatgerm, safflower, sunflower and soyabean oils), nuts and seeds, wheatgerm, asparagus, spinach, broccoli, butter, bananas and strawberries.

Beta Carotene

Beta carotene is the precursor to vitamin A and therefore functions in a different way. Beta carotene has to be converted to vitamin A before it can be used. Nonetheless, beta carotene is a powerful quencher of free radicals, so it is important to ensure adequate intake by eating green, leafy vegetables and carrots.

Minerals

High blood pressure is a major risk factor in heart disease. An effective way of lowering blood pressure is to increase your level of calcium, magnesium and potassium. However, magnesium deficiency has far more serious implications. It is thought that a number of people who die from heart attacks do not die as a result of arterial blockage but by coronary artery spasm which blocks off blood flow. A deficiency of magnesium has been shown to produce a spasm of the coronary arteries. Furthermore, magnesium has been found to be helpful in strengthening heart muscle and in the management of cardiac arrhythmia. It is interesting to note that while there is a low incidence of heart disease in Eskimos, attributed to the EPA present in fish oils, their diets are also high in magnesium levels.

Coenzyme Q10 (COQ10)

The heart is a highly efficient pump and it requires a continuous supply of energy from one heartbeat to the next. Coenzyme Q10, found in rice, bran, wheatgerm, soyabean and beef, is one of a family of substances essential for generating energy. Indeed, COQ10 is a necessary component of the process which releases energy from

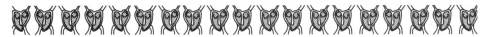

our food intake. The closest analogy is that of a spark plug in the body. Without Coenzyme Q10 there can be no spark and hence no energy. While COQ10 can be made by the body, recent reports suggest that as we grow older our bodies do not make enough of this life-generating nutrient.

Eating For A Healthy Heart

There appears to be little doubt that an increase in the incidence of heart disease, in common with other degenerative diseases, is linked to diet. Increasing our intake of fruits, vegetables and fibre and decreasing our consumption of saturated fats, coffee and alcohol will all help in reducing the risk factors. A recent WHO (World Health Organisation) report advocates a daily intake of 400 g of fruits and vegetables, to include pulses, seeds and nuts, to keep us healthy. The report also underscores the point that the typical Western diet is lacking in sufficient quantities of essential nutrients. There are reasons to believe that we may not be getting all the nutrients we need from our food, even if we are making the right food choices, and that we may be overfed yet remain undernourished.

Today's science of food manufacture may have produced cheap plentiful food, but on its way from the farm to the factory to the supermarket shelves, the food is depleted of vitamins and minerals. What little is left can be lost during its journey from the freezer to the microwave to the table. So although our food looks and possibly tastes the same as it did 50 years ago we cannot always be sure it will provide us with the nutrients we need.

What is more, artificial fertilisers, pesticides and crop sprays used in modern farming not only ensure that our food is grown with chemicals but is also covered in them – a further damaging effect on our health and well-being.

Thus, while proteins, carbohydrates and fats are generously provided by the diet, the more delicate micronutrients, such as vitamins and minerals, frequently are not. One way to ensure an optimum amount of micronutrients is by way of dietary supplements. These can be specially formulated mutivitamin mineral preparations that provide the recommended nutrient intakes as well as other dietary supplements, such as garlic, fish oil and lecithin, which are all beneficial for heart health.

General Guidelines For Healthy Eating

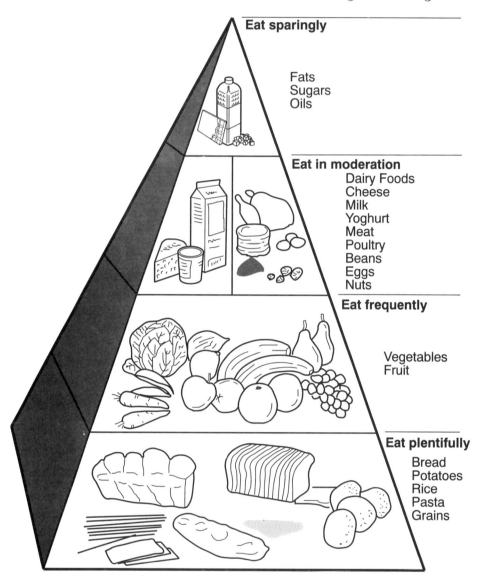

Eat sparingly

Fats
Sugars
Oils

Eat in moderation
Dairy Foods
Cheese
Milk
Yoghurt
Meat
Poultry
Beans
Eggs
Nuts

Eat frequently

Vegetables
Fruit

Eat plentifully

Bread
Potatoes
Rice
Pasta
Grains

The Healthy Eating Pyramid was evolved by nutritionists in the US. It has been adapted by the Dunn Nutritional Centre for application in Britain. It shows very clearly which foods we should be eating in large quantities and which we should be eating in only small amounts.

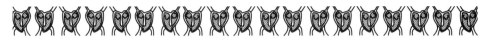

Supplements For Heart Health

- A broad-range multivitamin and multimineral formulation
- Vitamin C: 2 g per day
- Vitamin E: 200 iu per day
- Fish oils: 2 g per day
- Garlic: 1 g per day
- COQ10: 100 mg per day
- Lecithin: 3 g per day

Finding A Nutrition Therapist

Dietitians can be consulted free via your GP, as there is one in every district, usually based at the main hospital. Many are keen to help people improve their eating habits. Or, for a list of practitioners or further information write, enclosing a SAE to:

The British Naturopathic and Osteopathic Association, 6 Netherall Gardens, London NW3 5RR;

The British Society for Nutritional Medicine, 4 Museum Street, York, YO1 2ES;

The Nutrition Association, 36 Wycombe Road, Marlow, Buckinghamshire SL7 3HX.

Further Reading

A Healthy Heart For Life by Caroline Shreeve (Thorsons)
Conquering Heart and Artery Disease by Richard Brown (The Arterial Disease Foundation)
Heart And Blood Circulatory Problems by Jan De Vries (Mainstream Publishing)
Super Nutrition for A Healthy Heart by Patrick Holford (ION Press)
The Eskimo Diet by Saynor and Ryan (Ebury Press)
Vitamin Guide by Hasnain Walji (Element Books)
Vitamins, Minerals and Dietary Supplements: A Definitive Guide To Healthy Eating by Hasnain Walji (Headway)

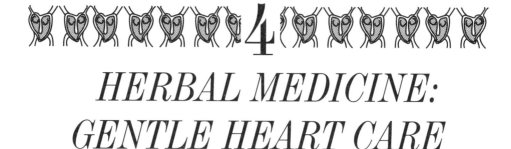

HERBAL MEDICINE: GENTLE HEART CARE

The ancient art of herbalism has been practised for thousands of years, and is still used today around the World. In fact, according to WHO it is the single most common method of healing.

What Is Herbalism?

Herbalism is the use of herbs and plants for healing. Many culinary herbs possess healing abilities but the variety of plants used for herbal remedies extends far beyond the selection which we use in the kitchen and includes flowers, mosses, seaweed, lichen and fungi. Herbal remedies draw on the many parts of the plant: the leaves, roots, seeds and even the bark may be beneficial. Also, different parts of the same plant may vary in their potency and effect: a skilled herbalist will know how to select the correct plant and the correct part of it to prepare a healing remedy.

A herbalist also needs to know the best method of administering the herb. Herbal remedies are prepared in a variety of ways – for internal or external use – according to the particular illness.

Internal Preparations

Decoction
A decoction is made from the roots or the bark of a plant. The plant is simmered for about 15 minutes, strained and drunk as a tea.

Infusion
This is a strong tea, like the decoction, but made from the leaves. The plant is simply made like an ordinary pot of tea. The leaves are left to 'stand' for about 10 minutes to allow the goodness to infuse into the water.

Tincture
This is a special herbalist method of preparation. Alcohol is poured over the herb, which is left to marinate for two weeks. After this

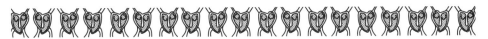

time, the mixture is decanted into a bottle, sealed and used as required. Tinctures are the most common form of herbal preparations used. Because they are concentrated only small doses are needed.

External Preparations

Ointment
The plant remedy is ground and usually mixed in an oily carrier base.

Compress
A compress is typically used on an open wound. A clean cloth is soaked in a hot decoction or infusion, and held firmly against the wound. The combination of the herb and heat is the key healing factor here.

Poultice
For a poultice, just the leaves of a plant are placed directly on the skin, wrapped in gauze. Sometimes a hot water bottle is held over the gauze. Sometimes a paste is made with dried herbs and applied with the gauze and heat.

Inhalants
The concentrated oil of a plant is placed on a handkerchief and inhaled (in the same way as the Victorians used smelling salts, for example), or burned over a candle in a special holder. This is aromatherapy — literally the 'therapy of aromas'.

How Does Herbalism Work?

Herbal remedies work with the body and act in three major areas:

- Elimination and detoxification: this is achieved through the use of *diuretics* (for increasing the flow of urine), *laxatives* (for loosening the bowels) and blood purifiers.
- Nourishment: this keeps the tissues, blood and organs in general overall good condition.
- Stimulation of the body's own healing abilities: the body's own natural functions are fortified and strengthened to withstand illness.

Conventional medicine can work against the body's natural functions: for example, the symptoms of a cold are the body's

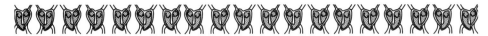

method of fighting off the infection (a raised temperature to kill the infectious organisms, sneezing and a runny nose to expel the toxins and tiredness to encourage the ill person to rest so that all the body's energy can be directed towards fighting off the cold). However, Western medicine prescribes cold remedies which are designed to suppress the symptoms of a cold and to keep us going about our everyday lives as if we were not sick.

Because herbal preparations are not isolated substances, the risk of side-effects is considerably reduced: other substances within the plant counteract the potential risk of the active ingredient. Nevertheless, herbs are powerful and, if used in the wrong way, can sometimes be toxic or harmful. Despite this, herbal remedies rarely cause side-effects, especially in comparison with conventional drugs.

The Holistic Approach

The difference between conventional medicine and herbalism is that herbalism takes a holistic – 'the whole' – approach. In practice this means that the underlying factors which produce the symptoms are treated. It is like taking a long-term instead of a short-term view. If a patient visits a GP with problems of indigestion, he or she is likely to be prescribed a digestive remedy which will cure the indigestion. A herbalist if confronted with the same patient would try to discover the cause of the indigestion and treat the cause as well as the symptoms of the indigestion itself. To do so, the herbalist would closely question the patient in order to build up a lifestyle profile: is stress the cause of the indigestion, or bad eating habits, or a biological disorder? Once the cause is discovered, the herbalist aims to create the correct conditions for the body to heal itself. Consequently, herbalist prescriptions are tailored to fit each person's requirements.

Whereas conventional medicine believes that the body needs a helping hand from synthetic drug preparations in order to heal, the herbalist considers that the body can heal itself naturally if the conditions for it are correct. Hence both emotional and spiritual well-being play their part in physical health.

Herbal medicine and orthodox medicine differ in their perception of 'good health'. In terms of conventional medicine, good health is simply an absence of disease; in holistic terms, good health is an absence of disease and a state of positive well-being. Herbal tonics can be taken on a regular basis to maintain good

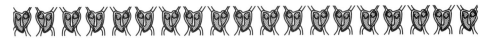

health and prevent disease; 'Prevention is better than cure' aptly describes the herbal approach to medicine. Conventional medicine, in contrast, is based on treating disease once it has already taken hold.

Today's Professional Herbalist

Western Medical Herbalists

A visit to a herbalist begins in much the same way as a visit to your GP: an examination is carried out which includes blood pressure, weight and pulse readings and listening to the heartbeat. Additionally, the herbalist will ask you questions about your diet, the amount of exercise you take, your drinking habits, family life and lifestyle. As well as prescribing a herbal medicine, suggestions may include advice on exercise and relaxation.

Chinese Herbalists

Yin and *yang* form the basis of Chinese philosophy and medicine. Basically, *yin* and *yang* are the direct opposites of one another and must both be present in order to maintain the natural balance. *Yin* is associated with cold, inactivity and darkness. *Yang* is associated with the opposite of *yin*: heat, movement and light. Ancient Chinese texts explain: 'If *yin* and *yang* are not in harmony, it is as though there were no autumn opposite the spring, no winter opposite the summer.'

In Chinese philosophy, humans and the environment are interrelated and so affect each other. If the balance between *yin* and *yang* falters, illness results. For example, if *yin* dominates, the result is exhaustion, passivity and weakness; if *yang* dominates, the result is irritability, excitability and hyperactivity.

Because of *yin* and *yang*, Chinese herbalism concentrates on maintaining the balance between the two aspects, and extends herbal remedies to the importance of warmth and coldness, movement and activity. A woman who has just given birth, for example, is recommended to only ingest hot foods and drinks, and to stay in the house for six weeks while she is given special herbal teas to fortify her and speed her recovery.

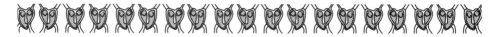

Types Of Herbs

Nervines

These act on the nervous system and are therefore useful for heart health. The nervous system can be overactive or underactive and there are herbal remedies to treat both of these accordingly. The nervine relaxants calm the system, the nervine stimulants stimulate it and the nervine tonics generally tone it up and keep it in good working order. For heart health, both the nervine relaxants and tonics are useful.

Carminatives

Carminative herbs act on the digestive system, encouraging it to eliminate toxins and absorb nutrients for the body's nourishment.

Diuretics

Diuretics encourage the production of urine and hence the elimination of toxins.

Tonics

There are tonics for the heart, just as there are for other parts of the body. These tone and strengthen the heart functions.

Herbal Remedies For Heart Health

Conventional medicine looks at the various heart problems and treats them separately. Herbalism, however, takes all the different heart ailments and treats them as one complaint: the holistic attitude rather than the separatist one. However, heart complaints are not suitable for self-medication. Consult a professional herbalist, as well as your GP/Consultant for advice and treatment.

Hawthorn Berries

These are a major herbal treatment for heart ailments. Hawthorn berries increase the blood flow of the heart, increase the force of contraction of the heart, lower high blood pressure, dilate the coronary arteries, reduce cholesterol levels break down fatty deposits in the artery walls and ease palpitations. The berries can be taken as an infusion or a tincture on a daily basis.

The addition of lime blossom and yarrow will further help the lowering of high blood pressure.

Garlic

Garlic, an all-round beneficial remedy, lowers blood pressure and reduces cholesterol. A great deal of scientific research over recent decades has proved the effects of garlic on health and, in particular, on heart health (see Chapter 3). The root itself can be taken on a daily basis (one clove) if you and your family are not averse to the pungent smell, or you can take garlic capsules. The Chinese name for garlic is *Suan*; the Chinese have used the herb for thousands of years.

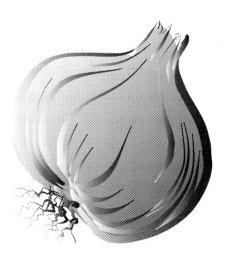

Garlic is not only a useful ingredient for adding flavour to your cooking, it will also help to keep you healthy.

Gingko Biloba

Gingko biloba comes from the gingko tree. It increases blood supply to the brain and helps prevent the build up of blood clots. Its use originated in Eastern medicine.

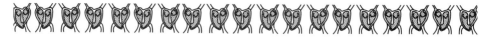

Ginger

Ginger has many uses but here we are concerned with its use in lowering cholesterol levels, opposing blood clotting and as an overall tonic to the cardiovascular system. An infusion or tea of ginger root can be taken, although some care is needed since ginger acts as a stimulant. Ginger in foods will be beneficial.

Broom

This increases blood pressure, has a diuretic effect and increases the pressure of each heart contraction. It is taken as an infusion or tincture on a daily basis. Broom is not suitable for self-medication – consult a professional herbalist.

Lime Blossom

This lowers blood pressure when used with hawthorn berries and is a good preventative against hardening of the arteries and hypertension. One of the nervine herbs, it is a relaxant, reducing stress and tension.

Valerian

Valerian lowers blood pressure and can reduce high blood pressure caused by stress.

Soyabeans

Soyabeans are used by the Chinese and are effective because of their lecithin content. Lecithin breaks down cholesterol if it is already present in high amounts; it also prevents the accumulation of cholesterol in a healthy person. Soyabean oil is taken daily or lecithin granules can be sprinkled on food. Lecithin is also available in capsule form.

Mistletoe

Mistletoe reduces high blood pressure, is effective in relieving hardened arteries, eases heart palpitations and relaxes the nervous system. Mistletoe is not suitable for self-medication – consult a professional herbalist.

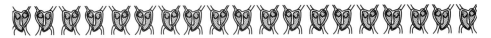

Yarrow

Combined with hawthorn berries and/or lime blossom, yarrow lowers blood pressure.

Caution If you are taking medicine from your GP or hospital consultant for a heart or circulatory problem, you should consult a professional herbalist before taking any herbal medicines.

Quick Reference Guide: Herbs for Heart Health

- Atherosclerosis: hawthorn berries, lime blossom, garlic, soyabeans, gingko biloba, ginger.
- High blood pressure: hawthorn berries, lime blossom, valerian, yarrow.
- Low blood pressure: ginger, rosemary.
- Hypertension: valerian, hawthorn berries, garlic, lime blossom.
- Cardiovascular diuretics: water retention caused by poor circulatory system (dropsy) can be relieved with yarrow, gingko biloba, dandelion leaf.
- Angina: hawthorn berries, lime blossom.
- Weak heart: a tonic of hawthorn berries, motherwort.
- Improving circulation: ginger, hawthorn, lime blossom, yarrow.

In addition to herbal treatment, attention to diet and exercise and ways of dealing with stress will be necessary for improved heart health. Herbal remedies are very efficient at preventing the onset of heart disease, but it is important that you consult a qualified practitioner before taking any herbal remedies.

Consulting A Herbalist

Western Medical Herbalist

A medical herbalist can give more specialist advice on the use of herbal medicine for serious or long-term problems. Medical herbalists undergo a four-year course at the School of Herbal Medicine and are trained to carry out general examinations. As a result of the overall diagnosis the herbalist will prescribe a single

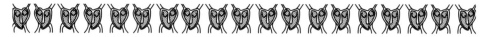

herb or combination of herbs and specify in which form the medicine is to be taken – as a tincture, as pills or as infusions.

Usually members of the National Institute of Medical Herbalists, these practitioners apply Western herbal medicine in a consulting room. The diagnostic techniques of many qualified medical herbalists resemble those of GPs, using the same methods and equipment for blood pressure, pulse taking, physical examination and assessment of urine and blood samples.

The National Institute of Medical Herbalists can be contacted at 9 Palace Gate, Exeter EX1 1JA.

Chinese Herbalists

Traditional Chinese herbalists tend to be confined to Chinese centres, practising mainly within the Chinese community. There is also the 'modern' practitioner of Chinese herbalism who uses herbs in conjunction with acupuncture.

The Register of Chinese Herbal Medicine can be contacted at 138 Prestbury Road, Cheltenham GLS2 2DP.

Ayurvedic and Unani Practitioners

Commonly known as *Vaids* and *Hakims*, these practitioners are mainly found within the Indian and Pakistani communities and offer treatment based on traditional principles.

Further Reading

A–Z of Modern Herbalism by Simon Mills (Diamond Books)
Herbal First Aid by Andrew Chevallier (Amberwood)
Herbalism: Headway Lifeguides by Francis Büning and Paul Hambly
   (Headway)
Herbal Medicine by Dian Dincin Buchman (Rider Books)
Secrets of the Chinese Herbalists by Richard Lucas (Lucas)
The New Holistic Herbal by David Hoffman (Element)
Traditional Home Herbal Remedies by Jan de Vries
   (Mainstream Publishing)

HOMOEOPATHY: THE VITAL FORCE FOR HEART HEALTH

Homoeopathy is based on the natural law *Similia similibus curentur*, which means 'Like cures like'. In other words, a disease can be cured by giving a substance which, if given to a healthy person, produces effects similar to the symptoms of that disease.

Homoeopathy is a holistic therapy which aims to go beyond the mere alleviation of symptoms to address the actual causes of ill- health. The ultimate aim of homoeopathic medicine is for the patient to reach such a level of health that there is no longer a need for, or dependence on, any medicine or therapy.

The therapy has its roots in ancient times. Homoeopathic principles are present in the writings of the fifth-century Greek physician Hippocrates, while the sixteenth-century Swiss alchemist Paracelsus commented that, 'Those who merely study and treat the effects of disease are like those who imagine that they can drive away winter by brushing snow from the door. It is not the snow that causes the winter but the winter that causes the snow.' Symptoms are not actually manifestations of a disease but rather the attempts of the body to heal itself.

Modern homoeopathy owes its establishment to the German physician Samuel Hahnemann. As a doctor in the late eighteenth and early nineteenth centuries, he was appalled at the way conventional medicine was practised. He considered the customs of bleeding patients, administering strong enemas and using powerful, and often dangerous, drugs to be both brutal and dangerous, evidenced by the high patient death-rate.

Hahnemann searched for a method of curing that was effective, safe and gentle. While translating Cullen's *Materia Medica*, Hahnemann was puzzled by the explanation for the efficacy of cinchona bark in treating malaria. He proceeded to dose himself liberally with cinchona bark for several days and developed malarial symptoms. In this way he established that, not only did cinchona bark alleviate the intermittent fever of malaria, but large doses of cinchona bark actually caused malarial symptoms in a normally healthy person.

Hahnemann went on to experiment with many other substances, testing them on himself, his family and friends. These experiments, called 'provings', involved the taking of very small doses of substances and carefully noting all the symptoms that were produced. Subsequently, patients suffering from similar symptoms were treated with the 'proven' substances; the results were encouraging and often remarkable.

Hahnemann's research led him to criticise conventional medicine, especially *allopathic treatment* (orthodox treatment of an illness with its opposite). Instead, he argued, the remedy for the healing of the disease should be one that artificially produces symptoms as similar as possible to those produced by the disease itself; 'Like cures like.'

The theory of homoeopathy developed, although not without opposition from the orthodox medical profession. Its value was particularly highlighted in the European cholera epidemics when many lives were saved by a homoeopathic prescription of camphor suggested by Hahnemann. By the time of Hahnemann's death in 1843, homoeopathy had spread over most of continental Europe and had penetrated Russia, South America, Great Britain and parts of the USA.

How Homoeopathy Works

The fundamental difference between homoeopathic and allopathic medicine lies in the way in which symptoms are viewed. While allopathic medicine views symptoms as being part of the disease, a homoeopath regards them as an adaptive response by the body in defending itself. Simply put, the symptoms are evidence of the body's fight against the disease. The homoeopath's task is to prescribe a remedy that will stimulate the body to heal itself more quickly. The correct remedy is one that will create symptoms similar to those of the disease process as presented by the patient.

Homoeopathy is based on the following three principles:

The Law Of Similars

The human organism is believed to have a great capacity to heal

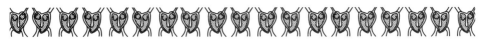

itself and is in a constant state of self-repair. The homoeopath prescribes a remedy which, through previous 'provings' on healthy people and from clinical observations, is known to produce a similar symptom picture to that of the patient. The prescribed remedy then stimulates and assists the body's own natural healing efforts.

The Single Remedy

Homoeopaths believe that the body should only be stimulated by a single remedy at any one time. It is the patient's whole system which is out of balance even though there may be a multiplicity of symptoms which may not appear to be connected. The single remedy allows the homoeopath clearly to observe and evaluate its effect before further prescription is considered.

The Minimal Dose

Only a minute dose, in the form of a specially prepared potency, is needed, since the patient is highly sensitive to its stimulus. This is because of the similarity between the remedy's known symptom picture and that of the patient. The specific potency and number of doses are determined by the homoeopath according to the needs of the individual.

Much debate and controversy surrounds the concept of dilution. As homoeopathic remedies are diluted to such an extent, sceptics say that it is inconceivable that any of the original substance is left at all, so how can such a remedy work? Homoeopaths would argue that, although they do not yet understand the mechanism, there is ample evidence that it does work.

Theories And Clinical Trials

Among the wide range of theories put forward to explain how homoeopathy works, one is the suggestion that looking for a physical explanation ignores the holistic nature of the therapy. It may well be the case that the high potencies are acting at a very subtle level of energy, as with *chi* in Chinese medicine or *prana* in Ayurvedic medicine, and that these remedies vibrate or resonate with a person's 'vital force'. The right homoeopathic remedy is like a boost of subtle energy which returns the body to its optimum frequency and so aids recovery. Once the body is in tune, resonating at its appropriate rate, it is able to use its immune system to throw

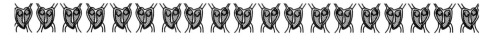

off the negative stimuli that cause illness.

There were many clinical trials in the late 1970s. One in particular, conducted in Glasgow in 1978, compared three groups of patients with rheumatoid arthritis. One group was told to take aspirin, another group a *placebo* (a non-medicated substance) and the last group homoeopathic medicines. A year after the commencement of the trial, the condition in the homoeopathic group was more significantly improved than in the two other groups.

Other trials conducted since then include David Reilly and Morag Taylor's hay fever trial in 1985, and Peter Fisher's fibrositis trial in 1986. In both of these, homoeopathic medicines were found to have a demonstrable effect in relieving symptoms. A recent study of over 100 clinical trials showed about 80 positive in favour of homoeopathic medicines.

The Homoeopathic Medicines

The range of sources for homoeopathic medicines is immense, since they can be prepared from anything that causes symptoms. Most come from plants but some come from metals and minerals. Today there are over 2,500 substances that have been prepared for homoeopathic medicines, from belladonna (deadly nightshade) and aconite (monkshood) to lachesis (an extract of snake venom) and cantharis (derived from the insect known as Spanish fly).

The medicines are made up by taking the raw material through a process of serial dilution and *succussion* (vigorous shaking). Each stage of succussion increases the potency, or strength, which is given a number and a letter. Potencies with an 'X' affix are diluted 1:9 and those with a 'C' affix are diluted 1:99 at each successive stage. Plant materials are instantly soluble, but minerals and metals need to undergo a process called *trituration* (grinding) with a milk/sugar powder up to the 3X potency before they become soluble; at that point the dilution and succession process continues in the same manner as plants.

Taking The Medicines

The remedy and potency prescribed are matched to the needs and vitality of the patient and also to the vitality of the disease process of the patient. The potency has to be similar in resonance to that of

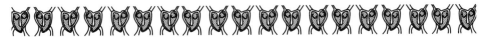

the disease, as well as similar to the symptom picture. Today there are many outlets which sell homoeopathic medicines over the counter, such as health food stores and pharmacies. They are available in tablet form, granules, pilules, powders or as a liquid, while there are creams, ointments and lotions for external use. It is usual for over-the-counter medicines to be of a lower potency, either 6C or 30C – caution is advised in the repetition of the 30C, as this is a relatively high potency. Higher potency medicines are generally recommended for use only by experienced and qualified homoeopaths.

The same medicine may be administered in different ways, perhaps a single dose in a high-potency form or a low dose repeated frequently. The choice of method depends on the nature of the illness and the individual needs of the patient. For example, if a person has been ill for a long time and the body is in physical disrepair, one way to take the homoeopathic medicine would be in repeated doses in a lower potency to stimulate the immune system. However, a healthier person may just need a single high-potency remedy for a response.

Dilution lessens the toxic effects of the substance used; this contrasts markedly with the powerful drugs often used in allopathic medicine, a number of which have been known to produce alarming side-effects. Further, since conventional drugs are prescribed for their individual capacities to work upon specific parts of the body, it follows that several different drugs might be prescribed to treat various symptoms in one individual. The effects of such combinations are often unknown or not recognised. A homoeopath, however, prescribes a single medicine in an appropriate potency which will stimulate a person's immune or defence mechanism and bring about an improvement in general health.

Homoeopathy And Heart Health

A homoeopath believes that symptoms like high blood pressure, anxiety and stress are a manifestation of the body's attempt to defend itself. Homoeopaths state that there are several levels of the body's defence systems. The first is eliminative: the body responds to stress or invasion by stimulating its defensive function without any conscious awareness by the person. Once this defensive response reaches a certain level, the body is able to feel the effects of its defence mechanism, giving rise to certain symptoms. Finally, when the body is no longer able to respond efficiently, it is open to chronic disease since it no longer has the ability to heal itself in its current state. Chronic conditions weaken the body's ability to deal with new threats and further decrease its ability to heal itself. The homoeopath will try to halt functional disorders and then to reverse them, all the while building up the body's strength and natural healing ability. The function of homoeopathy is to assist the body in maximising its defence potential as it tries to heal itself.

Whilst homoeopaths are happy for people to treat themselves in some cases of ill-health, such as for coughs and colds, for example, chronic conditions like heart disease must be treated by a professional. In these circumstances, homoeopathy can offer a long-term, safe alternative to treating heart complaints with orthodox drugs or surgery. Additionally, the homoeopathic consultation may well spot potential heart problems before they become dysfunctional, whereupon preventative action can be taken.

In Conversation With A Practitioner

Q. How long does treatment take?

A. This is a difficult question to answer, but after several interviews the homoeopath is better able to give you an idea of this. The nature of your complaint, its severity and how long you have been suffering from it, will all influence your body's ability to respond to treatment. Remember that arthritis and rheumatism in particular are chronic diseases which have taken a long time to develop: a quick cure is not, therefore, a realistic expectation.

Q. How many appointments are necessary?

A. During the first six months visits may be frequent but will taper off as you become healthier. We feel we need to see you initially more frequently (follow-ups are usually every four to six weeks in the beginning) to work with you and evaluate your progress. Yet we are not insensitive to the cost of treatment and do not wish to make this a burden. A happy medium can be reached.

If a remedy has brought your system into balance, in our experience this state can last for a long time. We would then need to wait until the next 'remedy picture' comes up clearly. This is the time to have renewed faith in your body's healing abilities.

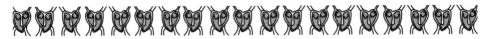

Q. How can I be involved?

A. You don't have to believe in homoeopathic remedies in order for them to work (we treat babies and there are homoeopathic vets). But to select the correct remedy and for the treatment to continue to act, your co-operation and commitment are necessary.

You can help by:

- Noting any changes after you take the remedy – keeping a weekly journal can be helpful for bringing to your follow-up consultations. Please note general changes as well as specific ones.
- Giving a clear and complete account of your symptoms on all levels.
- Above all, communicating any concerns or questions you may have. We are always trying to find better ways of helping you and welcome your comments.

Q. Where do I obtain my remedies?

A. We either have your remedy available at the clinic and will dispense it, the cost usually being included in your consultation fee, or we shall refer you to a convenient homoeopathic pharmacy.

Although there are over 2,000 remedies which are prepared in established homoeopathic pharmacies, most homoeopathic prescriptions are made from a narrower range of 200–300 remedies.

Q. Can homoeopathic treatment be undertaken at the same time as other alternative therapies, for example, acupuncture and chiropractic?

A. Following the principle of the single dose, we advise against other types of treatment while you are taking homoeopathic remedies. This is because we need to establish which remedies are successful and which are not: if you are receiving acupuncture at the same time, a homoeopathic practitioner will not know if it is his/her prescription which is resulting in any changes, or if it is due to the acupuncture. An acupuncturist would also prefer that you follow one type of therapy at a time. Similarly, essential oils can interfere with homoeopathy and should preferably be avoided while following a homoeopathic prescription.

Concerning chiropractic and osteopathy and their treatment while undergoing homeopathic treatment, we have found that mild manipulative therapy does not interfere with homoeopathy.

Q. Can a wrong remedy be given and what are the effects?

A. As much as we carefully try to match the correct remedy, we do not always achieve 100 per cent accuracy. If appropriately used, homoeopathic treatment should produce no side-effects from the remedies. Either nothing changes or the true symptom picture will become even clearer and the right remedy is more obvious.

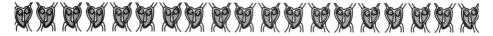

It can take several interviews for a homoeopath to get an accurate picture of the totality of your symptoms and an 'essential' understanding of this to select the right remedy. Of course, the clearer and more in touch you are with yourself the easier this task becomes.

Q. What about seeing a GP?

A. Homoeopathy is complementary to the health care that is available. We recommend you maintain your relationship with your doctor, especially for routine needs and emergencies. Your GP will also arrange for you to have any blood tests, X-rays, etc, or refer you to a consultant. It is also best to avoid, or at least greatly reduce, the intake of coffee and other caffeine drinks.

Q. What about seeing a GP?

A. Homoeopathy is complementary to the health care that is available. We recommend that you should maintain your relationship with your doctor, especially for routine needs and emergencies. Your GP will also arrange for you to have any blood tests or X-rays, etc, or refer you to a consultant.

Finding A Practitioner

An increasing number of qualified medical doctors now offer homoeopathic treatment. Most of them have taken a postgraduate training course to become a Member or a Fellow of the Faculty of Homoeopathy (MFHom or FFHom). A register of these is maintained by the Faculty of Homoeopathy, c/o Royal London Homoeopathic Hospital, Great Ormond Street, London WC1N 3HR. Many professional homoeopaths have trained for four years at accredited colleges and have become graduate or registered members of the Society of Homoeopaths (RSHom). For a list of registered homoeopaths, write to The Society of Homoeopaths, 2 Artizan Road, Northampton NN1 4HU.

In addition to the private and NHS practitioners, there are five NHS homoeopathic hospitals – London, Bristol, Tunbridge Wells, Liverpool and Glasgow. There are also a number of private clinics nationally. Further information about these may be obtained from The British Homoeopathic Association, 27A Devonshire Street, London W1N 1RJ.

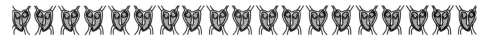

Further Reading

Everybody's Guide to Homoeopathic Medicines by Stephen Cummings
  and Dana Ullman (Gollancz)
Homoeopathy for Babies And Children: A Parents' Guide by Beth
  MacEoin (Headway)
Homoeopathy for Emergencies by Phyllis Speight (C W Daniels)
Homoeopathy: Headway Lifeguides by Beth MacEoin (Headway)
Homoeopathy, Medicine for the New Man by George Vithoulkas
  (Thorsons)
Homoeopathy: Medicine for the 21st Century by Dana Ullman
  (Thorsons)
The Complete Homoeopathy Handbook: A Guide to Everyday Health Care
  by Miranda Castro (Macmillan)
*The Family Guide to Homoeopathy: The Safe Form of Medicine for the
  Future* by Andrew Lockie (Elm Tree Books)

ANTHROPOSOPHICAL MEDICINE: ORGANISATION OF BODY WARMTH

Orthodox medicine is based upon hypothesis and experimentation; if something cannot be proven by experiment, it does not exist as a scientific fact. This premise can lead to an oversimplification, if it is applied to the physical aspect of existence only. Indeed, in conventional medicine (based on natural science) this simplification is a fundamental tenet, and we call it *reductionism*. All aspects of our existence – the physical, the manifestations of living organisms, the emotional and mental or spiritual aspects – are reduced to mere expressions of the physical.

In anthroposophical medicine, the methods and discipline of (natural) science are applied to other, non-physical levels of reality. Anthroposophy is also called a spiritual science; it acknowledges the other levels of our existence and investigates their inter-relationships. This approach broadens the possibilities of treatment of illness.

Anthroposophy was founded by the Austrian philosopher and scientist Rudolf Steiner (1861–1925); he outlined the philosophical foundations of his ideas in his treatise *The Philosophy of Freedom*. Steiner describes in this, and other works, how the human being has not just a body, but also a soul and spirit. He discerns four aspects to the bodily nature of the human being; health and well-being depends on a harmonious working together of these aspects.

Together with a Dutch doctor, Ita Wegman, Steiner further developed his ideas for medicine, and they wrote the book which marked the beginning of anthroposophical medicine: *The Fundamentals of Therapy*.

The Four Aspects Of The Human Being

In addition to the physical body, three other elements are present in the human body which complete the picture of the human being. In anthroposophical terms they are called the *etheric* (or life-)body, the *astral* (or sentient-) body and the *ego* (-body). These elements are

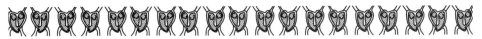

common to us all, but cannot be perceived directly by the ordinary physical senses. Essentially the *etheric* body is concerned with growth, repair and replenishment, the *astral* body represents the sentient and emotional life, and the *ego* embodies the individual spiritual core, which man alone possesses.

The Etheric Body

This is the force which governs the existence of the physical body. It imbues the physical body with life, without which the physical body deteriorates and disintegrates; this happens naturally after death, when only physical laws govern. The etheric body is responsible for keeping the physical parts of the body into a whole and maintaining its integrity by continuous repair and restructuring. It is the very source of our natural tendency to heal and recover from less serious ailments, without additional medical help. In short, the etheric body constantly guards against death and decay (physical laws).

The Anthroposophical Elements Of A Complete Person

Spirit	Self-consciousness	Human	Ego
Soul	Consciousness	Animal	Astral body
Life	Life	Plant	Etheric body
Material	Weighable and measurable	Mineral	Physical body

The Astral Body

The astral body represents the soul element, common to animals and humans, and differentiates them from the plants and minerals. Our sentient being, consciousness as such, is carried by the astral body.

It is through our sentient (astral) body, that we are aware of emotions, feelings, thoughts: a level which cannot be measured tangibly, but is very much a reality. A conventional doctor believes that this aspect of our existence is a mere manifestation of physical and chemical processes. An anthroposophical practitioner regards the sentient life and therefore the sentient (or astral) body as a reality, just as much as the physical.

The astral body has, generally speaking, a strong *catabolic* (breaking down) effect in the human body, and so has an opposite effect to the etheric body, which is constantly endeavouring to build

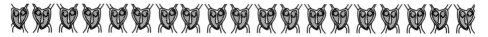

and repair. So, good health prevails for as long as the destructive (*catabolic*) processes, due to the activity of the astral body, are held in check and in equilibrium by the building (*anabolic*) activity of the etheric body. An imbalance between the two will result in illness.

The Ego

Present only in the human being, the ego adds an additional level of consciousness, namely the self-consciousness. It comprises the ability to think independently and brings an awareness of being autonomous. So humans are able to refrain from instinctive behaviour, if reasoning leads them: a quality that is not present in the animal world. The human ability to learn, develop and become an independent and lonely being, is due to the ego, the spiritual core of man. On a bodily level, this ego has quite a complicated task and influences, generally speaking, the etheric body in an anabolic way and joins the astral body in its catabolic activity. However, the ego always guards the totality of the bodily processes and works mainly through the warmth organisation of the body.

The Anthroposophical View of Illness

Anthroposophical practitioners look at health and illness in terms of the interrelationships between the ego, the astral body, the etheric body and the physical body. These four aspects of the human being interrelate and interconnect to each other in different parts of the body and its organ systems.

The three main functional organ systems within anthroposophical medical thought are described as the nerve–sense system, the metabolic limb system and the rhythmical system.

The nerve–sense system comprises, physically, the central nervous system (brain, sense organs, spinal cord) and the whole of the autonomous nervous system (connecting to all the internal organs).

This organ system lacks vitality, regeneration and movement. The nervous system is very vulnerable and easily damaged if deprived of oxygen and other nutrients. The life-bringing activity of the etheric body is therefore very minimal, and the catabolic action of the astral body dominates, bringing about consciousness, thought and perception.

In the metabolic limb system we find a wealth of vital activity in the main digestive organs (liver, pancreas, stomach etc.), the

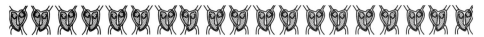

lymphatic system and our reproductive organs. The muscles of our limbs are the main consumers of nutrients and are full of life and movement.

There is no consciousness in this system and we are not aware of its anabolic processes, unless there is something wrong and we feel pain; pain is heightened consciousness, and is experienced through our astral or sentient body. The astral body also works in the metabolic limb system, but here not in a catabolic way. It serves the predominantly anabolic activity of the etheric body. Whilst in the nerve–sense system the catabolic activity overrules the anabolic.

The tension between the catabolic and anabolic processes in these two organ systems is regulated by a third functional activity–that of the rhythmical system.

The Three Systems In Anthroposophical Medicine

Nerve–Sense:	Thinking	Conscious	Cooling Catabolic Hardening
Rhythmic:	Feeling	Dream-like	Balancing Meditating
Metabolic Limb:	Volition	Unconscious	Warming Anabolic Softening

This rhythmical system of the body is found most clearly in the rhythmical activity of the heart, circulation and breathing: *systole* (contraction) and *diastole* (expansion), in-breath and out-breathing, illustrate the constantly changing balance of the rhythmical system. It incorporates and balances both the primarily catabolic action of the nerve–sense system (contraction, consciousness enhancing), and the mainly anabolic activity of the metabolic limb system (relaxation, regeneration).

Such a dynamic and artistic view of the functions of the human body enables the anthroposophical doctor to relate anatomical and physiological aspects to psychological and spiritual aspects in the human being. Illness and dis-ease result from imbalances in the interrelating systems. Such an understanding broadens the scope of diagnosis as well as treatment. Different methods of treatment are used to achieve this.

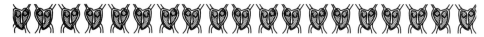

The Medicines

When and where appropriate and/or necessary, conventional medicines are and will be used. However, the remedies developed in anthroposophical medicine are derived from plant or mineral and, occasionally, animal sources. The choice of substance is based on the perceived relationship between the life process in the human body and nature. Steiner gave many indications of how certain substances relate to bodily processes and organs; for example, he indicated how the seven metals (lead, tin, iron, copper, mercury, silver and gold) correspond to organs and organ-processes. So an anthroposophical practitioner might prescribe a potentised preparation of tin, as drops or in the form of an ointment, for a patient with liver problems, or copper for regulation of the kidney function. Plant substances may well be given in material doses, as well as in potentised form.

Artistic Therapies

Artistic activity engages and appeals to the creative sources of the human being; the aim in therapy would be to mobilise such creative potential, and not particularly to create a work of art as such. Being engaged in a creative process also influences our bodily functions, in different and often subtle ways. Painting with a blue colour only will have a calming effect on our breathing and circulation, whilst sculpture work will engage our will more directly. For both physiological and psychological reasons, activities such as music, painting, form-drawing and sculpture may be recommended as part of an integral treatment plan.

Eurythmy Therapy

This therapy developed out of the art-form *eurythmy*, which Steiner also called *visible speech* or *visible music*. It is an art of movement (dance) through which the formative and creative forces of the world are made visible, in an artistic way. The eurythmy therapist uses specific gestures that express, for instance, certain vowels or consonants in a certain sequence. Through these movements, a soul-mood is created and they engender changes in the breathing, circulation and distribution of muscular tension. The exercises are used in the treatment of both physical and psychological disorders.

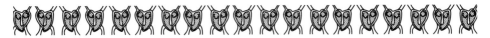

Hydrotherapy And Massage

In these treatments, the physical body is more directly addressed. A special form of rhythmical massage was developed, which in comparison with other forms of massage, is quite gentle. The masseur will identify patterns of muscular tension, warmth penetration and distribution, and the tone of the skin and underlying soft tissues. Particularly the irregularities of the warmth organisation are noted, as the warmth as such is regarded as the physical medium through which the activity of the ego works. Through addressing the warmth, with oil-dispersion baths and using particular aromatic oils in the massage itself, a self-sustaining improvement and redistribution of warmth and tension can be achieved. Particularly the rhythmical system is strengthened in relation to the other functional systems; the breathing relaxes and deepens, a healthier flow of warmth comes about, relieving inappropriate tensions.

The Treatment Of Heart Complaints

Since heart problems are so individualistic, the anthroposophical doctor will look at the person as an individual and make recommendations accordingly.

Finding A Practitioner

Anthroposophical practitioners are all qualified medical doctors who have taken a further postgraduate course recognised by the Anthroposophical Medical Association in Britain. Some may be found working in the NHS, although others work privately or in the Rudolf Steiner schools and homes for children in need of special care (Camphill Communities). Residential treatment is also available.

Consultations are very much like seeing a GP except that there may be additional details and questions about, for example, lifestyle and emotional situation. Diagnosis is made in the same way as a GP and treatment is prescribed depending on the individual characteristics of the patient.

Treatment will range from conventional, anthroposophical or herbal to homoeopathic types of medication. In addition, eurythmy, massage, hydrotherapy or an art therapy may be prescribed to

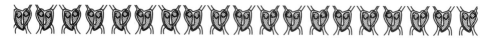

complement and enhance the treatment.

The Anthroposophical Medical Association maintains a register of members. It is based at the Park Attwood Therapeutic Centre, Trimpley, Bewdley, Worcestershire DY12 1RE.

Further Reading

Anthroposophical Medicine by Dr M Evans and I Rodger (Thorsons)
Anthroposophical Medicine and its Remedies by Otto Wolf (Weleda Ag)
Rudolf Steiner: Scientist of the Invisible by A P Shepherd (Floris Books)

7

ACUPUNCTURE, ACUPRESSURE AND THE ALEXANDER TECHNIQUE: RESTORING HARMONY

Acupuncture and acupressure are ancient Chinese healing therapies which are radically different from any Western healing practices. They are both founded on essential principles of Chinese philosophy which state that all living matter is activated by a life force, or energy, called *chi*. Without *chi*, life cannot exist. The life force is believed to flow along channels within the body which are referred to as *meridians*. Ill-health arises when the *chi* cannot flow freely: traditional Chinese medicine is entirely concerned with maintaining the flow of *chi* along the meridians.

The flow of *chi* is dependent upon the correct harmony of *yin* and *yang*. According to Chinese philosophy, everything in the human body, the World and the Universe has this dual aspect.

The Meridians

The major meridians, of which there are 12, are, apart from the *triple warmer*, named after the parts of the body to which they relate, that is, the *large intestine, stomach, heart, spleen, small intestine, bladder, circulation, kidney, gall bladder, lung* and *liver*. In addition, there are the *central* and *governing* meridians. Manipulation of points along the particular meridians is said to influence the *chi* and *yin-yang* balance.

Acupuncture

How Does Acupuncture Work?

The body's energy network is tapped into by inserting various needles at strategic points below the skin. There are some 800 acupuncture points which link to the 12 major meridians.

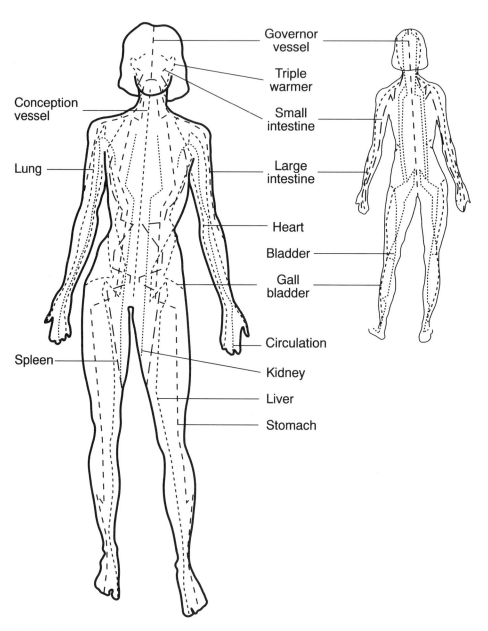

Governor vessel

Triple warmer

Small intestine

Conception vessel

Large intestine

Lung

Heart

Bladder

Gall bladder

Circulation

Spleen

Kidney

Liver

Stomach

The Meridians

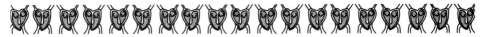

Scientific research has not found any evidence of the meridian channels, which in our Western world amounts to a condemnation of acupuncture as simply 'the placebo effect': the patient believes it will work and so it does. Yet acupuncture is a common form of treatment in the East to this day, and is used in the treatment of everyday ailments and as an anaesthetic in major operations. So how does it work?

One theory is that acupuncture encourages the body to release its natural painkillers, the *endorphins* and *enkephalins.* These painkillers are known to be effective in treating depression and allergies. This *anaesthetising* effect of acupuncture has also been attributed to the 'gate control' theory of pain: the theory that there are *neuropathways* to the brain via the spinal cord which, if blocked, cannot send messages of pain to the brain. While this may account for the anaesthetic effects of acupuncture, it does not explain acupuncture's success in healing non-painful conditions.

Another theory to explain the success of acupuncture takes into account the fact that pain in the organs or muscles is felt on the surface of the body – on the skin. This suggests that our bodies are indeed a complex network of sensory devices; once this precept is understood the concept of applying pressure to certain parts of the body for healing does not seem so strange after all.

Origins Of Acupuncture

The origins of the theory of *chi* lie in ancient China although it is unclear how acupuncture was discovered. It is claimed that about 4,000 years ago it was observed that warriors who were wounded by arrows miraculously recovered from diseases that had been troubling them for many years. It was also noticed that certain organs seemed to be associated with specific points on the body which often became tender when the body was diseased and that these points could be used for the treatment of disorders.

The original needles were made from stone and did not penetrate the skin; bone and bamboo needles did, but these were used later. Undoubtedly, a cause-and-effect relationship was worked out by noting the point punctured and the disease it cured. When metal was discovered, the needles were made from copper, silver, gold and other alloys.

The earliest written record dates from the time of the Yellow Emperor Huang Ti, who lived in the Warring States period in China

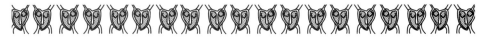

(475–221 BC), and has been reprinted in modern times as the *Yellow Emperor's Classic of Internal Medicine.*

Acupuncture was introduced to the West during the Ching dynasty (1644–1911) although the Chinese themselves attempted to ban it for political reasons. It reached Germany in the seventeenth century and then France in the middle of the nineteenth century. Due to pressure from the Western powers, which effectively ruled China at this time, the Chinese government again tried to ban traditional medicine in 1922, but its practice continued covertly until it was positively espoused by Chairman Mao in the aftermath of the Second World War when acupuncture treatment and research was given fresh impetus and energy.

Even today acupuncture has great grass-roots support. In China, especially, the motivation behind the promotion of acupuncture has been the relative poverty of the country and the lack of 'conventionally' trained physicians, drugs and medical equipment – but also because it works well in primary health-care situations. Indeed, acupuncture is used widely by the general population and needles and other equipment can be purchased in shops as easily as aspirin can be bought in the West.

The West's interest in acupuncture was initially fuelled by the writings of the French diplomat Soulie de Morant in the 1940s. Later, acupuncture was brought to the attention of the West during the presidency of Richard Nixon. While visiting Peking, to report on 'ping-pong diplomacy' the renowned American commentator James Reston contracted acute appendicitis which required immediate surgery. This was successfully carried out under local anaesthetic while the postoperative pain was treated with acupuncture. This so impressed him that he visited many other centres where acupuncture was practised and, on his return to the USA, he did much to focus both professional and public attention on this therapy.

A Visit To An Acupuncturist

Diagnosis is a complex affair. To begin with, the professional acupuncturist will require a full medical history and observe particular features, such as the appearance of the face, tongue and eyes, and the condition of the skin. Aspects such as the distinctive odour of the body, personal gestures and voice tone will assist the practitioner in making a diagnosis. But practitioners vary. Some also make a physical examination or include medical tests.

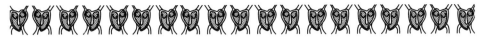

Next, the practitioner will take pulse readings from each wrist. This is quite different from Western pulse taking. Pulse diagnosis is an extremely skilled and complex matter which takes years to master and increasingly is not used by modern acupuncturists who do not subscribe to its use. The traditional acupuncturist, however, places the index, middle and ring finger of his right hand on the patient's left wrist and takes six readings which are described in one of 28 terms including 'weak', 'thin', 'light', 'tight', 'fine', 'hasty' and then does the same for the opposite wrist using his left hand. This exhaustive pulse diagnosis gives the practitioner an insight into the health of the person's individual organs, circulatory and immune systems and much more, and forms the basis of the prescription.

A detailed picture of the gravity of the disorder and energy flow can be obtained from the pulse readings.

After the diagnosis is complete, the acupuncturist decides which acupuncture points to manipulate for the restoration of the patient's energy pattern. Each point has a particular function attributed to it and groups of points can act like a 'combination lock' whereby the entire formula is more important than their relevant individual attributes. The most usual way to do this is with fine needles, usually made of stainless steel.

Acupuncture is not a simple affair and a qualified acupuncturist has taken years to master its skills. Recently the British Medical Association has issued warnings against acupuncturists, but this applies to cowboys who may only have taken a weekend course in acupuncture to learn the rudimentary pain-killing methods. It is always advisable to ensure that practitioners are suitably qualified and experienced: there are four professional bodies which are affiliated to the Council for Acupuncture which maintains a register of practitioners (see page 96).

The Use Of Needles

Most people's reaction to the thought of needles being put into them is one of total aversion. In fact, the sensation is said to be relatively painless, with only a slight tingling felt, provided the procedure is carried out expertly.

The needles are inserted vertically, obliquely or almost horizontally, usually only a fraction of an inch below the skin. Specialist treatment may call for different types of needle and deeper insertion may be required, although this is not considered to

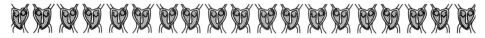

be any more painful than the shallower insertion. The needles are left in for a few minutes only or for up to half an hour, depending on the particular point and the ailment which is receiving treatment. The needles are rotated and manipulated to stimulate activity.

Moxibustion is a type of acupuncture treatment in which a ball of dried mugwort is placed on top of the needle's handle, the needle inserted and the herb set alight. Alternatively, the herb may be placed on the patient's skin, set alight and adroitly whisked away before any heat reaches the body. The needle is inserted afterwards. Some practitioners pass an alternating electrical current down the needle in order to identify acupuncture points: points are identified by decreased electrical resistance.

Auriculotherapy is another form of acupuncture which concentrates entirely on the ear. It is founded on the principle that all the body's parts can be affected by their correlation with the ear. This is based on the theory that the ear resembles the human foetus in its position in the womb (inverted with the head pointing downwards). Two hundred points on the ear have been found to be effective in acupuncture treatment. Auricular acupuncture is carried out with an electronic instrument which simultaneously detects the points and stimulates them; however, needles are often used. Some acupuncturists combine auricular acupuncture with general acupuncture.

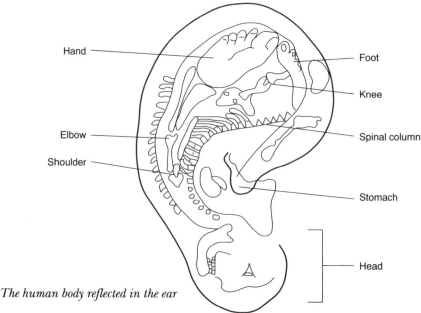

The human body reflected in the ear

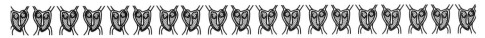

Acupuncture And Cardiovascular Health

Correctly administered, acupuncture, unlike drugs, will not leave any side-effects other than a feeling of relaxation. Treatment for cardiovascular health may include needles on the Lung and Circulation meridians. Auricular points which might prove beneficial are the Lung, Chest and Neck points. Taken together, stimulation of these points is likely to restore the balance of *chi* which has caused the disease. Stimulation along the Circulation meridian will improve blood flow and its pressure.

Otherwise, a general acupuncture course to strengthen the immune system, thereby maintaining a good circulation, would be beneficial as a 'Prevention is better than cure' tactic.

Acupressure

Acupressure is a combination of the techniques of acupuncture and massage. Acupressure is the art of using the fingers to press particular points (the acupuncture points) on the body to stimulate the body's own healing powers, rather than using needles.

When you have a headache and rub your temples you are employing acupressure to relieve the pain. Similarly, when you knock your elbow and rub it to ease the pain, that is also acupressure. It can be practised anytime, anywhere and by yourself. The only equipment needed are your own two hands. There are no side-effects and it is surely the most natural therapy available to us.

The Potent Points

The potent points are the same as the acupuncture points. Pressure applied to a potent point stretches the muscle fibres and improves the circulation of the blood. This aids the immune system and therefore increases the body's resistance to illness. Stimulation of the potent points releases endorphins. When endorphins are released not only is pain sensitivity blocked but oxygen flow increases; this enables the muscles to relax.

There are three types of potent points:

- *Local point.* This is the actual area where pain or discomfort is felt. Application to the local point will bring relief.
- *Trigger points.* These points work by triggering a reflex in another part of the body. The triggering mechanism is believed to be effective because

the stimulus is carried through the meridians.

- *Tonic points.* These are points which are effective in the maintenance of good health. A popular tonic point is in the webbing between the thumb and the index finger.

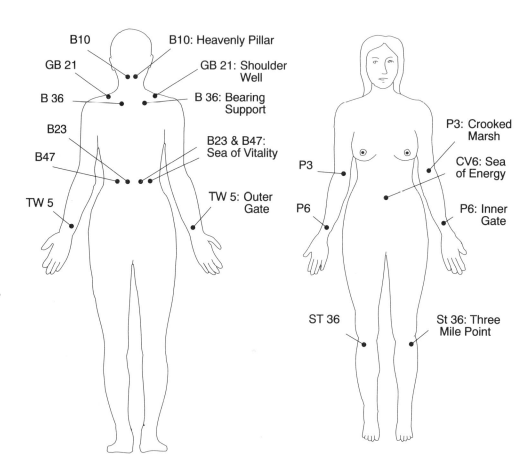

Locating The Points

Each point has two references. The original ancient Chinese name tends to describe the benefits felt from the point. For example, Shoulder Corner eases shoulder pain, while Three Mile Point is supposed to give a person sufficient energy to run 3 miles! This point has been used effectively by athletes to increase stamina and endurance. Additionally, each point has a number which is universally used by practitioners of acupuncture and acupressure.

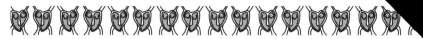

The points can be located by reference to anatomical features such as bone indentations. Some points lie in a knot in a muscle and the skill of the practitioner lies in correctly locating the points. This is important for the specific management of certain conditions.

Practising Acupressure

There are four main types of pressure: firmly, slowly, brisk rubbing and quick tapping.

Pressure is applied for just a few seconds if the intention is simply to tone and stimulate the circulation. If there is pain, pressure should be maintained for several minutes. Stiff muscles can be eased by using slow, kneading movements. Brisk rubbing increases circulation, tones the skin and relieves chills and numbness. Quick tapping with the fingertips is for tender areas, such as the face, and improves nerve functioning.

Ideally, you should practise acupressure on a daily basis, for an hour at the most, but two or three times a week will also be beneficial.

Acupressure For Cardiovascular Health

- The potent point Heavenly Pillar (B 10) relieves tension. It is at the base of the skull, about half an inch out from the spine.
- Shoulder Well (GB 21) not only relieves shoulder tension but also tiredness, irritability and anxiety. Pregnant women must be careful when applying pressure to this point.
- Crooked Marsh (P 3) eases chest pain, as does Inner Gate (P 6). Crooked Marsh is just inside the elbow, while Inner Gate is located on the forearm, just a little bit up from the wrist. The easy availability of these potent points makes it very easy to apply pressure wherever and whenever is convenient.
- The potent point Bearing Support (B 36), found in the shoulder blade, is described in ancient Chinese writings as a preventative against colds and 'flu. Bearing Support is taken to be especially useful in boosting the immune system, as are Three Mile Point (St 36), Sea of Energy (CV 6), Sea of Vitality (B 23 and B 47) and Outer Gate (TW 5).

The Alexander Technique

Teachers of the Alexander Technique believe you can learn to improve your posture so that your body is able to work in a more

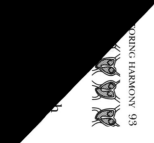

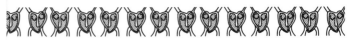

...nd efficient manner. The technique is entirely
...rmonious state of both mind and body, and
...hing mechanism, which means there is less
... heart. The heart lies within the ribcage so any
rigidity, or hyperventialtion as a result of anxiety, can reflect on its
functioning.

The Alexander Technique was developed by an Australian actor,
Frederick Matthias Alexander, who found himself losing his voice on
stage and discovered that he could cure the problem by improving
his posture. He realised that the relationship between the head,
neck and back was vitally important for good health. His discovery
became the basis for a whole technique for retraining the body's
breathing patterns and movements. Today there are Alexander
training schools and teachers all over the world, helping people find
a more efficient way of living, thereby putting less stress on the body.

Learning The Technique

'Lessons' are usually given on a one-to-one basis. The 'teacher'
begins by watching how you use your body. Even simple activities
such as walking or reading a book involve the use of many muscles,
and a certain amount of muscular tension and 'spring' is needed
just to react against the pull of gravity. Children move naturally, but
so often acquire bad habits as they grow up. Stress and holding the
breath is evident in such simple actions as grasping a pen too tightly
or clenching the jaw while concentrating. If we hold our breath we
can begin literally to squeeze the life out of ourselves. We slump
down in front and put extra pressure on the heart. We make life
difficult for ourselves and this lack of ease is often the forerunner to
disease.

Medical science realises that the attitude of the patient plays a
very important part in the recovery process. Through the Alexander
Technique, you can take control and positively re-establish the ease
which you have lost. The Alexander Breathing Pattern is vitally
important in this process.

Glynn Macdonald, a highly experienced teacher of the Alexander
Technique and author of *The Alexander Technique* (Headway), writes,

> 'Stand in front of the mirror and gently blow the air
> out through your mouth. Watch your upper chest and
> shoulders and check that they do not move too much.
> There will be a little movement, but your chest should

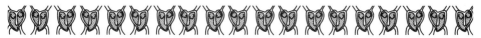

> remain fairly balanced and stable. Allow your head to nod gently forward. At the end of each breath, shut your mouth and notice how the air comes back in through the nostrils. Do not sniff the air in, as this will narrow the nasal passages and restrict the amount which gets into the lungs. Sniffing may mean you are taking your breath in forcibly, rather than trusting that it will come in naturally.'

Some people suffer from chronic muscular tension, which throws the head, neck and back out of alignment, causing rounded shoulders, a bowed head, stiff joints and arched back. If this is not corrected, the spine develops a curve, and a hump may appear at the base of the neck. This causes back pain and puts a strain on the heart, lungs and digestive system. Breathing can be restricted and poor circulation can develop. If you correct these problems of posture, the heart has a chance to operate more efficiently.

The Alexander teacher shows you how to stop these harmful habits and begin to use muscles with minimum effort and maximum efficiency. While you stand, sit or lie down, the teacher gently manipulates your body into a more efficient and effective way of being, while explaining to you where you are going wrong. Gradually, by constant practising and thinking about how you perform even the simplest actions, you should learn to release tension and use your body correctly. The teacher uses no force and there is no wrenching or clicking of joints – just a subtle adjustment as you learn to walk, sit, stand and move all over again, in a free, released way. Your breathing improves and your essential Breath of Life is given enough space to operate.

Lessons last about 30 or 45 minutes, and a course of 30 is usual, after which you should have learnt the basics.

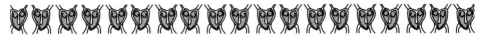

Finding A Practitioner

Acupuncture and Acupressure
The fact that anyone can call themselves an acupuncturist makes it all the more important that you establish that the practitioner is properly trained. There are four professional bodies which are affiliated to the Council for Acupuncture, 38 Mount Pleasant, London WC1X OAP, which maintains a register of practitioners. They are the British Acupuncture Association and Register, the International Register of Oriental Medicine UK, the Register of Traditional Chinese Medicine and the Traditional Medicine Society.

Alexander Technique
For information about the Alexander Technique, contact the Society of Teachers of the Alexander Technique (STAT) 10 London House, 266 Fulham Road, London SW10 9EL.

Further Reading

Acupuncture by Alexander Macdonald (George Allen & Unwin)
The Acupuncture Treatment of Pain by Leon Chaitow (Thorsons)
Acupressure's Potent Points by Michael Reed Gach (Bantam Books)
Alexander Technique: Headway Lifeguide by Glynn Macdonald (Headway)
Acupressure: Headway Lifeguide by Eliana Harvey and Mary Jane Oatley (Headway)

8

AROMATHERAPY: HEARTSCENT HEALTH

The fragrance of a rose. Bath bubbles which 'contain herbs to help you relax, leaving you refreshed and revitalised'. Pot-pourri to fill your home with a pleasing fragrance. A gentle massage which leaves you feeling relaxed and toned. What do these have in common? They all contain elements which, taken together, form the practice of aromatherapy: the combination of the powerful effects of touch and smell.

Aromatherapy uses the essential oils of plants to beautify, relieve stress and alleviate a variety of ailments. It is a practice which dates back to the ancient Egyptians, who used the powerful healing effects of aromas in their medicine. When Tutankhamun's tomb was opened 70 years ago there still lingered traces of the frankincense and myrrh which were used for his mummification and which were buried with him for his use in the afterlife. The Romans used plant essences in their temples, their homes and for medicinal purposes, and it is thought that it was they who introduced the practice of aromatherapy to Britain. The Chinese have left records from 1000–700 BC which describe how they also used plant essences for culinary, medical and cosmetic purposes.

While the Middle Ages saw a decline in rational medicine in Europe, in Asia it flourished. Abu Ibn Sina, an Arab born in 980 AD and known in the West as *Avicenna,* was a leading physician of his time. He is credited with the development of the technique of distillation which is still used for the preparation of essential oils to this day. But is was not until the Renaissance that Europeans once again started to investigate medicine and with it the healing power of herbs and their essential oils. At this time, antiseptics, perfumes and medicines all came from herbs.

The Industrial Revolution during the nineteenth century heralded the age of chemistry and chemical substitutes brought a decline in the use of plants and their essences until it was found that these substitutes were not effective in the same way as their natural models. (Each essential oil is a complex mixture of organic

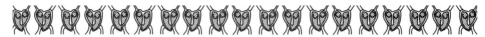

substances, and its therapeutic value depends on not just one of its constituents, but on the whole delicate mixture. The number of constituents in essential oil make it impossible to make exact chemical copies.)

It was not until a French doctor, René Gattefosse (1881-1950), accidentally discovered the healing power of lavender oil that aromatherapy was reborn. Working in his laboratory one day, he burned his hand and plunged it into the nearest available liquid, which happened to be essential lavender oil. When his hand healed extremely rapidly and without trace of a scar, he was intrigued by the therapeutic effects of lavender oil. His subsequent research led to the widespread use of aromatherapy, even to the extent of its usage to heal wounded soldiers during the First World War. The name *aromatherapy* was coined by Gattefosse.

After Gattefosse's death, his work was continued by the French physician Jean Valnet who used essential oils of clove, lemon and chamomile as natural disinfectants and antiseptics to fumigate hospital wards and to sterilise surgical instruments. The link between aromatherapy and the cosmetic industry was forged and developed by a French biochemist, Marguerite Maury (1895-1968), who was instrumental in developing the aromatherapeutic massage techniques.

Extracting The Essential Oils

Essential oils are extracted from all parts of the plant – from leaves and flowers, roots, seeds and rinds. There are various extraction techniques. The most common is steam distillation where steam is passed under pressure through the plant material and the heat causes the release and evaporation of the oil. The oil then passes through a water cooler where it condenses and is collected.

Some oil is extracted from flowers using solvents. In this case, a solvent such as petrol ether is sprayed over the flowers and this extracts the oil. The solvent is evaporated off, leaving the oil. Citrus fruits are a much simpler affair: pressure is applied to the rind and the oils are collected in a sponge and then simply squeezed out.

The quantity of plants required to produce essential oils is staggering: 70 kg of plants yield, on average, just 1 kg of essential oil. This can vary according to the season and even the time of the day that the plant is harvested – jasmine is harvested at sunset to yield the greatest amount of oil from the flower, while rose has so little oil

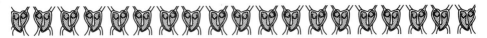

that it may take 100 kg of some varieties of rose petals to make half a litre of oil. The final price of the essential oil depends on yield, which is why rose is one of the most expensive of the essential oils. (Other expensive oils are melissa, jasmine, lovage, neroli, etc., depending on harvest conditions.)

How Does Aromatherapy Work?

It is not entirely understood how aromas affect our moods, but there is no dispute that they do. One theory is that the area of the brain which is sensitive to smell is close to the area which deals with emotions, memory and intuition (the *limbic* area) and as a result smells can affect the way we feel. On safer ground, it is known that all essential oils have some powerful antiseptic qualities. Most also stimulate the immune system, with the result that they encourage the body to resist disease and alleviate pain.

Essential oils are absorbed into the body via the blood stream. This can be via the skin (during massage, in a bath or on a compress) or via inhalation (through a diffuser, or a few drops on a handkerchief, or in a bath).

The benefits of massage are, of course, more clear-cut. It provides manipulation on specific areas which require treatment, relieving pain in the muscles and joints. It stimulates the immune system and improves the circulation of the blood and the lymph system. Not to be overlooked is the overall effect of a good massage in promoting relaxation and easing stress. Touch is an important medium through which to express love. From birth, through childhood into adulthood, touch is the basic, physical means of communicating affection, giving comfort and instilling a sense of security.

Aromatherapy massage aims to treat the whole person, to restore both physical and emotional well-being.

Holism And Aromatherapy

Holistic treatment treats the whole of the body and not only the affected part. Further, it treats not just on a physical level but also on emotional, mental and spiritual levels. If you have a headache, for example, you will have the physical symptoms of raised blood pressure. You could simply take a drug to lessen this blood pressure. A holistic remedy would look to why the blood pressure was raised: was it a symptom of a circulatory problem? Or was it caused by stress

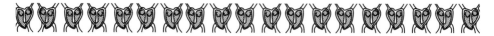

and, if so, what kind of stress? Holistic medicine gets to the root of the problem and deals with that rather than quashing the symptom and leaving matters there. The aim is to prevent a recurrence of the problem by taking appropriate health steps in the beginning.

Aromatherapy has become widely practised during the last few years, with aromatherapy oils readily available. But the current emphasis is mainly on aromatherapy's role in beauty therapy and as a relaxant. A professional aromatherapist, however, possesses clinical knowledge and can treat skin diseases, pre-menstrual syndrome (PMS), post-natal problems, headaches and circulatory problems, in addition to relieving stress and promoting a feeling of physical well-being.

A Visit To An Aromatherapist

A professional aromatherapist needs general medical knowledge in order to correctly diagnose a health problem. Consequently, a visit to a practitioner will begin with an overall assessment of your health. Close questioning to assess your eating habits, the amount of exercise you take and your general state of health will aid in a tailor-made prescription for you. After all, it is no use prescribing a remedy for a stress-related headache, for example, if the cause is in fact a food allergy!

Some aromatherapists prescribe essential oils for their patients, others allow the patient to make the choice, believing that the body should be trusted to choose what it needs. Having chosen the necessary essential oils, the next step is to decide how they should be administered.

Administering Essential Oils

The most potent method of administering the essential oils is by inhaling them. A few drops are placed on a handkerchief and inhaled, taking deep breaths. The oils pass directly into the system via the olefactory nerves to the brain and thence throughout the body. Alternatively, a few drops of the oil added to a bath will promote relaxation with the added soothing effect of the warm water. True aromatherapy, however, combines the benefits of the essential oils with the benefits of massage. The oil(s) are mixed with a base oil (sunflower or almond oil, for example) and massaged into the body. In this way the oils pass through the skin directly into the bloodstream.

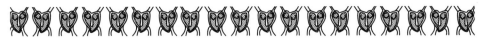

A practitioner may recommend a single course of treatment (usually six sessions), or further courses, or a continuation of treatment by yourself at home, depending on your ailment and your rate of recovery.

Aromatherapy Massage

To enhance relaxation, every attention is given to create the right atmosphere for a massage. A purpose-built massage couch ensures the comfort of the recipient of the massage and of the therapist giving the massage. The room will use colour – pastel shades of green, blue or peach or pink – to promote a sense of well-being; strong reds or black tend to exude energy rather than relaxation. The room temperature will be warm – no-one can relax if they are cold. There may be flowers, an essential oil burning, perhaps some relaxing music, and soft lights. If you are giving a massage to someone else in your home you should seek to create a similar environment, and also ensure that there will not be any interruptions which would break the relaxing atmosphere.

The oils are never poured directly on to the skin, but rubbed into the masseur's hands first. The spine, limbs and face will be worked on, although not the eyes as the eye tissue is very delicate and would be irritated. The professional aromatherapist will try to sense feelings of energy which are emitted from parts of the body, and where there is pain to 'draw' it out. Sometimes there are crystals in the massage room as it is believed that crystals can 'soak up' harmful energies and dispense healing ones. Particular attention will be paid to giving an overall feeling of relaxation as this helps the body's own healing systems to function better. This is especially important in cases where high blood pressure is a problem. Since massage encourages the circulation, aromatherapy treatment is especially beneficial for cardiovascular problems.

Aromatherapy At Home

Your aromatherapist may recommend that you continue the treatment at home. This may be by way of foot or hand baths, a compress on a painful limb, or perhaps simply burning essential oils using a diffuser.

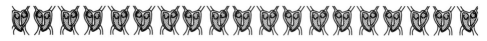

Essential Oils For Cardiovascular Health

Against Angina

- It may be surprising to hear that for angina a stimulant is recommended: the essential oil of black pepper, in fact. This essential oil is also beneficial for hypotension and as a general tonic for the circulation. It can be used in these contexts in a massage, in a bath or as a compress.

Against Atherosclerosis

- Juniper has many benefits for cardiovascular health. It encourages the circulation and used in massage and baths is effective in encouraging the breakdown of accumulated cholesterol deposits. This is because it is a general blood purifier and detoxifier. It also has a calming effect and will ease stress.
- Lavender is an extremely versatile essential oil for cardiovascular health – its properties as a detoxifier and stimulant to the circulatory system are beneficial when used in massage and baths.
- Neroli is a general blood purifier and cardiovascular tonic.
- Lemon and rosemary are blood purifiers and therefore beneficial in atherosclerosis.
- The uses of garlic oil in lowering cholesterol levels have been well documented and are explained in detail in Chapter 3.

Against High Blood Pressure

- Lavender can relieve high blood pressure because of its calming, sedative qualities.
- Lemon and rosemary regulate blood pressure and so are beneficial either in high or low blood pressure problems.
- Ylang ylang is effective in lowering high blood pressure, because of its generally sedative effect.

Against Low Blood Pressure

- Lemon and rosemary regulate blood pressure and so are beneficial for either low or high blood pressure.

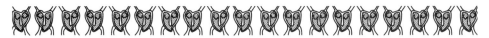

Against Arrhythmia

- Lavender, because of its sedative effect, can soothe palpitations. Rosemary also soothes palpitations, as do garlic and ylang ylang.

Against Stress

- Lavender has a very calming, relaxing effect: it used to be put inside pillows to encourage a good night's sleep. A few drops in the bath will soothe.
- Marjoram and chamomile are both relaxing and uplifting: chamomile tea has been a favourite on the Continent for centuries.
- Neroli is not only an antidepressant but also calms tension and stress.

In Conversation With A Practitioner

Q. Can aromatherapy be used to treat all types of illnesses and conditions, or are there limitations?

A. This is a difficult question to answer, as it varies not only from practitioner to practitioner but from country to country. In France, for example, doctors use aromatherapy for a variety of ailments, and even prescribe essential oils for internal use – in the same way as conventional doctors use drugs.

In this country, though, the majority of aromatherapists are not medically trained, so they tend to concentrate on aromatherapy as a means of reducing stress, which in itself can trigger a healing effect. This is just my approach, although other aromatherapists would say, yes, aromatherapy can treat any condition. In theory, aromatherapy can be used to treat any illness.

Q. Can anyone treat themselves using aromatherapy, at home, even for quite serious illnesses?

A. I wouldn't say serious illnesses, no, you would need help from a holistic practitioner who would take an overall look at your illness and your whole lifestyle – otherwise you are just treating the illness symptomatically which would never really do much. For instance, if you have athlete's foot you can put lavender oil on it and it may go away, but on the other hand it may come back again – in which case you're never actually doing anything to address the cause which may be not just the effect on feet of being

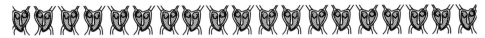

enclosed in trainers, perhaps, but a symptom of stress, vitamin B deficiency, whatever. There may be a need for deeper treatment: a look at the diet, taking garlic capsules, perhaps. You can treat minor ailments at home but if it doesn't work, and keeps coming back it may be necessary to look deeper.

Q. Can aromatherapy be used safely in conjunction with other therapies, such as acupuncture, homoeopathy and with conventional drug treatment?
A. With acupuncture, I don't think there is a problem, although again this depends on the practitioner. Some acupuncturists would say that it's best if you just have one treatment at a time, otherwise you don't know if the treatment is working. Otherwise, I think that gentle massage with a very low dilution of oil wouldn't do any harm at all – and I think it would be harmonious, because it's all about balance.

  With homoeopathy, again, some homoeopaths are very strict about using any aromatics – even toothpaste will act as an antidote to some of the remedies, whereas some homoeopaths disagree, so there really isn't any definitive answer. But traditionally eucalyptus and peppermint, and perhaps camphor, have been known to antidote oils as does coffee, simply because it is so aromatic. It's best to ask the homoeopath. I very much doubt that doctor's prescribing conventional drugs would object to their patients receiving an aromatherapy massage.

Q. As a practising aromatherapist, would you be happy for a patient to undergo homoeopathic treatment or acupuncture at the same time as taking essential oils?
A. Yes, as long as not too many treatments are mixed at the same time. Massage in general is such a good relaxant it enhances the internal conditions which help to trigger our immune defences.

Q. Talking about massage, it wasn't until this century that massage was introduced as a part of aromatherapy treatment – how crucial is it to aromatherapy?
A. Before Marguerite Maury's use of massage in the 1950s doctors tended to use essential oils as simply another form of herbal medicine to treat external conditions. Mood enhancing herbs were used by the ancient Egyptians but not as essential oils because techniques of distillation among the ancients were not yet discovered.

  In France doctors do not use massage very much – Maury brought the technique to this country. Massage is about the most important part of the therapy in this country as a means of relieving stress and this is the

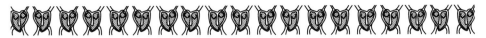

area which most interests me. Most illness is the result of disharmony of the emotions and the mind.

Q. In this country essential oils are commonly available: are there any guidelines to purchasing oils?
A. The best is to know the oils with a practised nose, so that you buy the pure essential oils; very often they are too diluted for traditional dosages to benefit. Buy from well-established herbal houses or from reputable health food shops.

Q. Would you ever prescribe oils to help people with emotional problems, for example, frankincense is reputed to help a person to cope with change and to move on?
A. No. Bach Flower remedies are useful for this but not essential oils. Response to aromas is very subjective and you just can't predict how a person is going to react to a particular oil. What you can predict is whether the aroma can uplift or relax but not the detail of whether it will stop you procrastinating. Maybe they do help but there is no specific evidence in this sphere. The citrus oils are cheerful but not if you don't like their smell!

Q. How do the essential oils boost the immune system?
A. They release endorphins which make us feel happy. But all pleasures in life have this effect. Of course, when we are happy we are less likely to become ill. Thyme, chamomile and lavender are widely used in France to boost white cell production. Aromatherapy is a multifaceted therapy which works on many levels. It boosts our own healing mechanisms on a physical and emotional level.

Q. Are there any conditions which must not use essential oils, for example, serious heart conditions?
A. Provided there are no allergies, I would give the patient oils which are not contra-indicated to smell and see if the reaction is favourable or not.

Q. How much experience is necessary to use essential oils?
A. If you have no experience, keep to very low concentrations and avoid the known potentially risky oils – clove oil is one which should never be used directly on the skin, for example. It's a matter of being sensible.

Q. How would I go about finding an aromatherapist?
A. The International Federation of Aromatherapists keeps a list of qualified practitioners which is a good starting point and word of mouth is the best recommendation. You need to find an aromatherapist you get

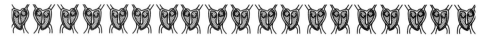

on well with — you just won't respond to someone you dislike, in the same way that you need to like your GP — after all, you won't relax if you don't like the aromatherapist who is giving you a massage.

Q. Where do you place aromatherapy in the field of healing?
A. In my opinion, aromatherapists should only see themselves in a complementary field, that is, to aid the person's own healing mechanisms and to promote relaxation, and not to say that you can treat chronic diseases outright.

Q. What would you say is the most important healing aspect of aromatherapy?
A. The tender loving care which an aromatherapist provides.

Finding An Aromatherapist

There are increasing numbers of weekend courses in aromatherapy and you should ensure that the aromatherapist you propose to consult is properly qualified and not just someone who has completed one of these introductory courses. Apply to one of the two following registered bodies who maintain registers of qualified aromatherapists.

International Society of Professional Aromatherapists, Hinkley and District Hospital, The Annexe, Mount Road, Hinkley, Leicester LE10 1AG

International Federation of Aromatherapists, 46 Dalkeith Road, Dulwich, London SE21 8LS

Further Reading

Aromatherapy by Daniele Ryman (Piatkus)
Aromatherapy : A Definitive Guide to Essential Oils by Lisa Chidell (Headway)
Aromatherapy for Everyone by Robert Tisserand (Arkana)
Aromatherapy: Headway Lifeguides by Denise Brown (Headway)
Aromatherapy – Massage With Essential Oils by Christine Wildwood (Element Books)
Massage: Headway Lifeguides by Denise Brown (Headway)

9

CONCLUSION

Heart attacks are the body's most extreme form of making us stop and evaluate our lifestyle. A heart attack shows that we have been taking things to extremes and not giving ourselves the time, care and attention which we need to avoid ill health. By 'taking things to extremes', I mean too much concentration on one area of life: perhaps too much time at work at the expense of family and friends; perhaps an intense concentration on work as a means to avoid repressed anger and strong emotions. The heart is traditionally the seat of our emotions and perhaps a heart attack shows that the emotions have been dammed up for too long. It may show that we are out of touch with our physical and emotional needs; an obsession with getting ahead ignores the non-materialistic and inner aspects of our being, to the detriment of the natural rhythms of life.

Of course, a heart attack may have a purely physical cause, most likely connected with poor diet – we need to give ourselves time, care and attention when thinking about our diet, as well as when thinking about our emotional health.

The first moment that you notice poor circulation, from cold hands or feet, is the moment to stop and consider why your body is failing. Blood is the life-giver: it contains the nutrients and oxygen which our body needs and it relies on the good health of the heart to be circulated. Any illness of the heart, the blood or the vessels through which the blood flows can be seen as a blockage of emotions, a failure to recognise them and allow their flow. Ask yourself, why you should deny your emotions, your inner self; why should you be concerned only with the purely physical, material world. Is extremism ever acceptable or beneficial? It is best to look at the whole picture with fresh eyes.

A heart problem, therefore, may not simply be a matter of constricted arteries or other purely physical problems such as high blood pressure or high cholesterol levels; it is a classic example of a body–mind interaction.

Does it make a difference which of the therapies, orthodox or complementary, you choose to attain health and well-being? There is no simple answer to this. If you are looking to eliminate the symptoms of your disorder as opposed to healing yourself, then any

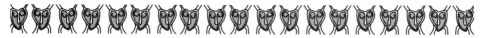

therapy that quickly and effectively deals with the symptoms would be acceptable. However, if you consider healing as attaining health and being wholly well again, then you have to look at all the therapies in a very different light.

Neither the GP and his drugs, nor the herbalist and her herbs, nor the aromatherapist and his essential oils, nor the acupuncturist and her needles, nor the osteopath and his manipulation, and not even the anthroposophical doctor with her art therapy, eurythmy and hydrotherapy can heal. Only you can heal yourself. 'Each patient carries his own doctor inside him,' said Dr Albert Schweitzer.

In order to begin the process of healing you must want to achieve health. The will to get better is paramount and consequently the body–mind interaction comes into play. A cognisance of this body–mind interaction will result in an integration of the body and the mind in the process of achieving wellness. That is what healing is all about. If this is understood, then it is easy to understand why the holistic therapies described in this book can be effective. However, whatever therapy we may choose, it can only be effective if we have a positive attitude towards the healing technique and the person who helps us to heal ourselves.

The culture of dependency spawned by modern medical intervention, of curing the sick parts of the body, has conditioned us to lose faith in our own ability to heal ourselves. We have come to rely on medication as a form of reassurance and believe that the prescription will 'cure'.

The root of this thinking is attributed to René Descartes whose dictum, 'I think therefore I am', crystallised the concept of separating *res cognitas* (the realm of the mind) and *res extensa* (the realm of matter). His perception of the material world has so permeated our culture that we now view the human body as an elaborate machine made up of assembled parts.

Descartes said, 'I consider the human body as a machine. My thought compares the sick man and an ill-made clock with my idea of a healthy man and a well-made clock.' This legacy of reductionism has guided and moulded the basis of modern medicine up to the present time.

Indeed, the study of disease has focused on biological processes, attributing the causes of all illness to biological factors. Modern medicine, preoccupied with measurements, statistical models and double-blind crossover studies, fails to take into account the person as a whole and appears to preclude the human potential for

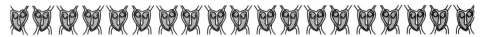

self-healing. The mind–body relationship has been ignored in healing. Whatever the disease, unless we accept that this relationship does exist, it is not possible to achieve true healing or true health and well-being.

We must first recognise that mind and body are both aspects of the human whole; that they are interrelated and cannot be seen in isolation from each other. The state of perfect balance between mind and body, as experienced in childhood, can be achieved. To do this, we have to understand how the mind and the body work together and affect each other.

There is a complex system of information that conveys messages between the mind and the body contained in our bloodstream. Regulation by the *pituitary gland* and the *hypothalamus* (a region of the brain situated between the eyes which has nerve connections from all over the nervous system) controls the psychological and emotional activity in relation to the physical function of the body. A good example of such a connection is the *vegas nerve* which links the stomach to the hypothalamus, hence stress or anxiety can cause stomach upsets.

We have seen that the immune system is indispensable for defence against disease-causing substances. However, we can be left vulnerable to disease if certain hormones are released by the adrenal glands which disrupt the relationship between the brain and the immune system. In addition to stress, this disruption can be caused by repressed feelings such as prolonged anger, bitterness and other negative emotions and thoughts.

The *limbic system*, a ring shaped area in the brain, consists of clusters of nerve cells, including the hypothalamus. Called the 'seat of emotions', the limbic system regulates the *autonomic nervous functions*, such as sweating, digestion and heart rate, and has a bearing on our emotions and sense of smell. The limbic system is therefore important in the body–mind relationship. This, in turn, is influenced by the *cerebral cortex* (the part of the brain responsible for thinking, perception, memory and all other intellectual activity). Stress is an example of the result of the alarm bells sounded by the cerebral cortex when it perceives a life-threatening situation. As soon as the alarm bells ring, the limbic system and consequently the nervous system and the immune system are all galvanised into action. The reaction is tense muscles, constricted blood vessels and other symptoms that set into motion a general nervous disarray.

Some reactions are instantaneous, such as blushing; others, such

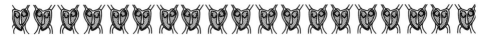

as repressed anger, are cumulative and take longer to manifest themselves in the form of disease.

There is little doubt that there is an innate link between the mind and the body, each affecting the other. Negative thoughts and emotions will result in weakened defences which will lead to disease and, ultimately, death. Our recognition of the body–mind connection is reflected in our everyday language when we say, 'He is eaten up with jealousy', or 'His heart is broken', or 'The stress is killing him', or 'He is worn down with grief', or 'She is radiantly happy'.

Most of the traditional healing disciplines, based on different world views and cosmological principles, all have a common thread: they deal with illness by considering humans in the context of their relationship with the cosmos.

The Yogic view of the human body is that it is composed of three different manifestations, namely, the physical body (composed of flesh, blood and bone), the subtle body (containing the life force *prana*) and the spiritual body (which encompasses universal wisdom).

To the Hawaiians, health means energy. Good health is a state of *ehuehu* (abundant energy) and poor health is *pake* (weakness). Illness is caused by *mai* (tension) and healing is equated to the restoration of *lapau* (energy). Health therefore is 'a state of harmonious energy'.

The American Indians consider that *Earth Mother* is a living organism, and that all creations on this earth contain a life force and are part of a harmonious whole. Illness occurs when this balance is upset and the purpose of healing ceremonies is to restore both personal and universal harmony.

Tai Chi is the Chinese way of increasing the energy flow in the body and strengthening the body's resistance to disease. Tai Chi is thought to stimulate the kidney (seen as the life force energy) and to maintain vitality of mind, body and spirit.

Rudolf Steiner, the founder of anthroposophy (see Chapter 6), sought to go beyond the idea of healing the body. His acute perception led him to explore the spiritual side of existence and this resulted in an understanding of the ways of stimulating the natural healing forces in the person. Healing was a matter of considering the interrelation between the four aspects of the human being (the physical body, the etheric body, the astral body and the ego) and treating them as a whole.

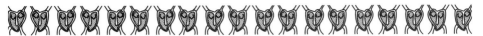

There are striking similarities in these healing systems. Call it by any name – *prana, rooh, chi*, life force, *ehuehu*, etheric energy – we all have it in us . It is up to the 'doctor inside', to borrow Albert Schweitzer's phrase, to harness this healing force within us and so to achieve that state of balance between body, mind and spirit.

Of late the holistic model of health care has begun to gain momentum. The proponents of this model have gone some way to counter the mechanistic and reductionist streaks in modern medicine. Holism is based on the premise that the human organism is a multidimensional being, possessing body, mind and spirit, all inextricably linked, and that disease results from an imbalance either from within or from an external force. The human body possesses a powerful and innate capacity to heal itself by bringing itself back into a state of balance. The primary task of the practitioner is to encourage and assist the body in its attempts to heal itself. The practitioner's role is that of an educator rather than an interventionist.

You picked up this book because you are concerned by the state of your own heart or that of a loved one and because you have an open mind, you are willing to explore different types of interaction between the body and the mind. **You** are responsible for drawing spirit into the equation and the final message of this book is that so-called 'holism' that looks only at the mind and the body, ignoring the spirit, is an illusion – go for a truer reality and use this book as, perhaps, a first step on the road to uniting body, mind and spirit.

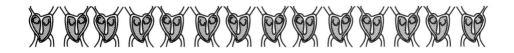

GLOSSARY

Acute   Symptom that comes on suddenly, usually for a short period.

Adrenaline   Hormone released by the adrenal gland, triggered by fear or stress.

Allergy   A condition caused by the reaction of the immune system to a specific substance.

Allopathy   A term used to describe conventional drug-based medicine.

Amino acids   A group of chemical compounds containing nitrogen that form the basic building blocks in the production of protein. Of the 22 known amino acids, 8 are considered essential because they cannot be made by the body and therefore must be obtained from the diet.

Anaemia   A condition that results when there is a low level of red blood cells.

Analgesic   A substance that relieves pain.

Antibiotic   A medication that helps to treat infection caused by bacteria.

Antibody   Protein molecule released by the body's immune system that neutralises or counteracts foreign organisms.

Antidote   A substance that neutralises or counteracts the effects of a poison.

Antigen   Any substance that can trigger the immune system to release an antibody to defend the body against infection and disease. When harmless substances like pollen are mistaken for harmful antigens by the immune system, allergy results.

Antihistamine   A chemical that counteracts the effects of histamine, a chemical released during allergic reactions.

Antioxidants   Substances which inhibit oxidation by destroying free radicals. Common antioxidants are vitamins A, C, E and the minerals selenium and zinc.

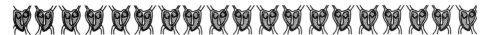

Antiseptic A preparation which has the ability to destroy undesirable micro-organisms.

Artherosclerosis A disorder caused when fats are deposited in the lining of the artery wall.

Atopy A predisposition to various allergic conditions like asthma, hay fever, urticaria and eczema.

Auto-immune disease A condition in which the immune system attacks the body's own tissue e.g. rheumatoid arthritis.

Autonomic nervous system Part of the nervous system which controls the involuntary and autonomic function of organs. It consists of a network of nerves divided into two parts: the sympathetic nervous system and the parasympathetic nervous system.

Benign Non-cancerous cells; not malignant.

Beta carotene A plant substance which can be converted into vitamin A.

Bile Liquid produced in the liver for fat digestion.

Candida albicans Yeast-like fungi found in the mucous membranes of the body.

Carcinogen Cancer-causing substance or agent.

Cartilage Connective tissue that forms part of the skeletal system, such as the joints.

Chi Chinese term for the energy that circulates through the meridians.

Cholesterol A fat compound, manufactured in the body, that facilitates the transportation of fat in the blood stream.

Chronic A disorder that persists for a long time; in contrast to acute.

Circulatory system Comprises of the heart and blood vessels; responsible for maintaining a continuous flow of blood in the body.

Cirrhosis Liver disease caused by damage of the cells and internal scarring (*fibrosis*).

Collagen Main component of the connective tissue.

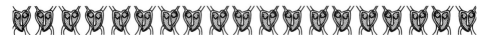

Constitutional treatment Treatment determined by an assessment of a person's physical, mental and emotional states.

Contagious A term referring to a disease that can be transferred from one person to another by direct contact.

Corticosteroid Drugs used to treat inflammation similar to corticosteroid hormones produced by the adrenal glands that control the body's use of nutrients and excretion of salts and water in urine.

Detoxification Treatment to eliminate or reduce poisonous substances *(toxins)* from the body.

Diuretic Substance that increases urine flow.

DNA A molecule carrying genetic information in most organisms.

Double-blind placebo controlled trials A type of trial to compare the benefits of a treatment where neither the patients nor the doctors know which patients are receiving treatment and which are on a placebo – an inert substance given in place of the drug/ treatment being tested.

Elimination diet A diet which eliminates allergic foods.

Endorphins Substances which have the property of suppressing pain. They are also involved in controlling the body's response to stress.

Enzyme A protein catalyst that speeds chemical reactions in the body.

Essential fatty acids Substances that cannot be made by the body and therefore need to be obtained from the diet.

Free radicals Highly unstable atom or group of atoms containing at least one unpaired electron.

Gene marker Indication of a particular gene defect, in a specific fragment of DNA, determined in laboratory tests.

Hepatic Pertaining to the liver.

Histamine A chemical released during an allergic reaction, responsible for redness and swelling that occur in inflammation.

Holistic medicine Any form of therapy aimed at treating the whole person – mind, body and spirit.

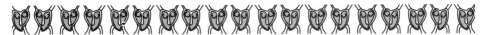

Lymphocyte A type of white blood cell found in lymph nodes. Some lymphocytes are important in the immune system.

Malignant A term that describes a condition that gets progressively worse, resulting in death.

Meridian Energy pathways that connect the acupuncture and acupressure points and the internal organs.

Mucous membrane Pink tissue that lines most cavities and tubes in the body, such as the mouth, nose etc.

Mucus The thick fluid secreted by the mucous membranes.

Myocardium muscle Special type of muscle that makes up much of the heart; contracts automatically and rhythmically when given sufficient oxygen.

Neurotransmitter A chemical that transmits nerve impulses between nerve cells.

Oxidation Chemical process of combining with oxygen or of removing hydrogen.

Pacemaker A small electrical device connected to the heart with an electric wire to supply electrical impulses to maintain the heartbeat.

Parasympathetic nervous system Also part of the autonomic system, the parasympathetic nervous system is concerned with the body's everyday functions, such as digestion and excretion. It slows down the heart-rate and stimulates the organs of the digestive tract.

Placebo A chemically inactive substance given instead of a drug, often used to compare the efficacy of medicines in clinical trials.

Potency A term used in homoeopathy to describe the number of times a substance has been diluted.

Prostaglandin Hormone-like compounds manufactured from essential fatty acids.

Sclerosis Process of hardening or scarring.

Stimulant A substance that increases energy.

Sympathetic nervous system Part of the autonomic nervous system, primarily concerned with preparing the body for action in times of stress or excitement. It stimulates functions such as heart-rate, sweating and increased blood flow to the body.

Toxin A poisonous protein produced by disease-causing bacteria.

Vaccine A preparation given to induce immunity against a specific infectious disease.

Vitamin Essential nutrient that the body needs to act as a catalyst in normal processes of the body.

Withdrawal Termination of a habit-forming substance.

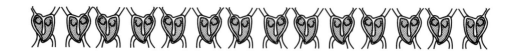

INDEX

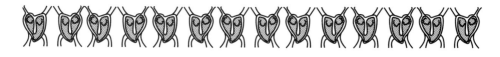

THE NATURAL MEDICINES SOCIETY

The Natural Medicines Society is a registered charity representing the consumer voice for freedom of choice in medicine. The Society needs the support of every individual who uses natural medicines and who is concerned about their continued existence in order to achieve the necessary changes needed to accomplish their wider availability and acceptance within the NHS.

The Society's aims are to improve the standing and practice of natural medicine by encouraging education and research, and by co-operating with the government and the EC on their registration, safety and efficacy. A major drawback in this work has been that none of the Department of Health's licensing bodies has any experts from these systems of medicine sitting on their committees – this has meant that not one of the natural medicines assessed by them has been judged by anyone with an understanding of the therapy's practice. Since the formation of the Society, it has worked towards the establishment of expert representation on the committees appraising these medicines.

To fulfil these aims, the NMS formed the Medicines Advisory Research Committee in February 1988. Known as MARC, its members are doctors, practitioners, pharmacists and other experts in natural medicines. It is the members of MARC who undertake much of the necessary technical and legal work. They have discussed and submitted proposals to the Department of Health's Medicines Control Agency (MCA), on how the EC Directive for Homoeopathic Medicinal Products can be incorporated into the existing UK system, and how medicines outside the orthodox range can be fairly evaluated.

The EC Directive for Homoeopathic Medicinal Products was eventually passed as European law in September 1992, incorporating anthroposophical and biochemic medicines, as well as homoeopathic. With discussions regarding the implementation of

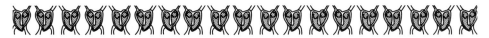

the Homoeopathic Directive now in progress, the MARC's work begins in earnest.

In July 1993, the MCA sent out their consultation paper regarding the implementation of the Directive, which incorporates many of the suggestions submitted by MARC. In it they propose to set up a committee of experts to advise on the registration of homoeopathic, anthroposophic and biochemic medicines. This is a major step forward for the Society, and homoeopathy in general.

With MARC members becoming increasingly involved in the legislative process of the implementation of the Directive, the Natural Medicines Society can now move forward from the short-term aim of protecting the availability of the medicines, to the longer-term aims of promoting and developing their usage and status by instigating and supporting research and education. The NMS has already sponsored some research – it is important to stress here that the Society does not endorse, support or condone animal experimentation – including an expedition to the rain forests in search of medicinal plants, supporting a cancer research project at the Royal London Homoeopathic Hospital and contributing to a methodology Research Fellowship. On the educational side, the Society has published two booklets, with several more planned and has co-sponsored a seminar for doctors and medical students.

The Natural Medicines Society depends upon its membership to continue this unique and important work – please add your support by joining us.

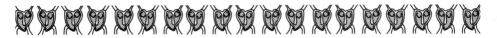

IF YOU ARE NOT ALREADY A MEMBER WHY NOT JOIN THE NATURAL MEDICINES SOCIETY?

(BLOCK CAPITALS PLEASE)

Mr/Mrs/Miss/Ms _____

Address _____

_____

Postcode _____ Tel. No. _____

There is no 'fixed' annual membership fee. Please indicate below the amount you wish to pay: minimum £5 (students and unwaged); European countries £15; non-EC £20.

£5 _____ **£10** _____ **£15** _____

N.B. Pay by Deed of Covenant and/or Direct Debit if you can—please ask for details.

Donations and offers of practical help are also always welcome to aid our fight to return natural medicines to the mainstream of medical practice.

I enclose a donation of £ _____

Please return this form with your remittance (cheques and PO's payable to The Natural Medicines Society), to:

**THE NMS MEMBERSHIP OFFICE,
EDITH LEWIS HOUSE,
ILKESTON,
DERBYS,
DE7 8EJ.**

(Registered charity no.327468)

You will receive your Membership Card, Member's Handbook, Quarterly Newsletter.

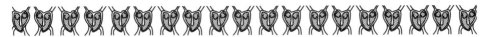

Author Profiles

Hasnain Walji is a writer and freelance journalist specialising in health, nutrition and complementary therapies, with a special interest in dietary supplementation. A contributor to several journals on environmental and Third World consumer issues, he was the founder and editor of *The Vitamin Connection – An International Journal of Nutrition, Health and Fitness,* published in the UK, Canada and Australia, focusing on the link between health and diet. He also launched Healthy Eating, a consumer magazine focusing on the concept of a well-balanced diet, and has written a script for a six-part television series, *The World of Vitamins,* shortly to be produced by a Danish Television company. His latest book, *The Vitamin Guide- Essential Nutrients for Healthy Living,* has just been published, and he is currently involved in developing NutriPlus™: a nutrition database and diet analysis programme for an American software development company.

Dr Andrea Kingston MB ChB, DRCOG, MRCGP, DCH is a Buckinghamshire GP in a five-doctor training practice who has for some years been interested in complementary approaches to healthcare as well as psychiatry and Neuro-linguistic Programming. Hypnotherapy is her major interest, and she has used this technique to help patients throughout the last eight years. As a company doctor to Volkswagen Audi, she contributes regular articles to the company magazine, *Link.* In the past, she has served as a member of the Family Practitioners Committee and as the President of the Milton Keynes Medical Society.

Books by the same authors in the Headway Healthwise series:
- Skin Conditions
- Asthma & Hay Fever
- Headaches & Migraine
- Alcohol, Smoking, Tranquillisers
- Arthritis & Rheumatism

Headway

Your Health in Your Hands

HEADWAY LIFEGUIDES

Simple and practical introductions to complementary therapies for the complete beginner.

Tai Chi
0 340 60008 X
£8.99

Alexander Technique
0 340 59680 5
£8.99

Herbalism
0 340 56575 6 £7.99

Aromatherapy
0 340 55950 0 £7.99

Homoeopathy
0 340 56578 0 £7.99

Massage
0 340 55949 7 £7.99

Reflexology
0 340 55594 7 £7.99

Shiatsu
0 340 55321 9 £7.99

Yoga
0 340 55948 9 £7.99

PUBLISHING SEPTEMBER 1994

Visualisation
0 340 61107 3
£6.99

Acupressure
0 340 61106 5
£6.99

HEADWAY HEALTHWISE

Self-help guides to managing common problems using integrated complementary and orthodox approaches. Endorsed by The Natural Medicines Society.

NEW SERIES

Asthma and Hay Fever
0 340 60558 8

Skin Conditions
0 340 60559 6

Alcohol, Smoking, Tranquillisers
0 340 60561 8

Headaches and Migraine
0 340 60560 X

Arthritis and Rheumatism
0 340 60563 4

Heart Health
0 340 60562 6

£6.99 each

Headway is an imprint of

Hodder & Stoughton
A MEMBER OF THE HODDER HEADLINE GROUP